PSYCHOGERIATRICS

A Practical Handbook

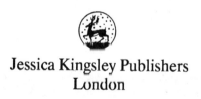
Jessica Kingsley Publishers
London

First published in Great Britain in 1989 by
Jessica Kingsley Publishers
13 Brunswick Centre
London WC1N 1AF

First published in Canada in 1987 by Gage Educational Publishing Company.

British Library Cataloguing in Publication Data
Psychogeriatrics by Donald A. Wasylenki
   1. Old persons. Mental disorders.
   I. Wasylenki, Donald A.
   DDC 618.976-89

ISBN 1 85302 037 0

Printed and bound in Great Britain by
Biddles Ltd, Guildford and King's Lynn

PSYCHOGERIATRICS

A Practical Handbook

to be returned on or before
below.

Donald A. Wasylenki, M.D., M.Sc., F.R.C.P.(C)

Head, Continuing Care Division
Clarke Institute of Psychiatry
Associate Professor, Department of Psychiatry
Faculty of Medicine, University of Toronto
Program Consultant, Community Psychogeriatric Service
West Park Hospital

Barry A. Martin, M.D., F.R.C.P.(C)

Consultant, Community Psychogeriatric Service
West Park Hospital
Head, Epidemiology and Biostatics Research Section
Clarke Institute of Psychiatry
Associate Professor, Department of Psychiatry
Faculty of Medicine, University of Toronto

Deborah M. Clark, B.S.W., C.S.W., M.Ed.

Director
Community Psychogeriatric Service
West Park Hospital

E. Anne Lennox, R.N., B.Sc.N., M.P.H.

Clinical Nurse Specialist
Geriatric Psychiatry Service
Queen Elizabeth Hospital

Lynda A. Perry, M.S.W., C.S.W.

Former Director, Community Psychogeriatric Service
West Park Hospital

Mary K. Harrison

Former Director, Community Psychogeriatric Service
West Park Hospital

Foreword

Psychogeriatrics: A Practical Handbook is addressed to physicians, nurses, and all other health and social service professionals who treat elderly people. The authors, who are practising professionals and leaders in community psychiatry for the ageing, give us the benefit of their experience. They suggest practical ways to help elderly persons affected by various mental health problems and also ways of giving support to their families and caregivers. Their relatively straightforward, rational but sensitive approach has helped many patients and families to avoid unnecessary admission to hospital or to a long-term care institution. However, their experience is as equally applicable in hospitals and chronic care facilities as it is in home-care programs and other settings in the community

The life expectancy of North Americans is now among the best in the world. In Canada, it is over 71 years for males and over 78 years for females. The fact that people are living longer has been noted in the scientific literature and in the public media. Generally, this achievement is not greeted with enthusiasm but by predictions of excessive dependency and economic burden in spite of the fact that the majority of old people consider themselves well and are actively involved in society.

The negative image of ageing derives, in part, from our literature. As noted in the preface, the deficits and disabilities that may occur are graphically described by Shakespeare, but they apply to a minority of elderly persons or to extreme old age, and are increasingly recognized as due to disease conditions rather than the ageing process. Ageing does produce decrements, but these chiefly reduce reserve capacity for dealing with excessive demands and need not limit the enjoyment of ordinary living. It is the high prevalence of chronic disease conditions, which characteristically appear in later life, that has made disability and dependency appear inevitable. We lack the knowledge of their causes and we cannot as yet prevent or cure most of them. However, the distinction of diseases of later life from the ageing process itself enables both clinicians and researchers to focus on the prevention, cure and/or more effective treatment of these diseases. In the absence of adequate knowledge at present, and for the benefit of persons now afflicted with these disease conditions, future research must also focus on ways of relieving distress, encouraging independence, and supporting the caregivers.

The quality of life of some older people may be seriously reduced by pain or disability, or by cognitive deficits that reduce the person's resilience and competence. These losses of health may be coupled with losses of spouse and children, and losses of income security and suitable housing. It is remarkable that old people generally can, and do, maintain a hopeful outlook and an interest in the lives of those dear to them. In a substantial minority, however, depressive reactions to loss and depressive psychiatric illness do occur and suicide rises with age. Social contacts and supportive interaction are vitally important to sustain someone experiencing such losses. Health professionals must be able to identify depression and provide the appropriate treatment. Psychological resolution of the loss by grieving is an important process that may require facilitation through sensitive help, not necessarily requiring a highly trained professional. The professional, however, can help those involved in the grieving process, or may take a more active therapeutic role if the underlying psycho-dynamics is understood. Throughout this book, the authors have given appropriate emphasis to the many losses experienced by the geriatric population. Those losses are addressed in such a way that very practical advice for the amelioration of suffering emerges from the text.

A major difficulty for professionals is to decide what is normal in physical and mental function for an older person. Each person is unique in genetic inheritance, and a lifetime of experience causes old people to become even more individualized. This, and the fact that research on ageing is in its infancy, means that we do not have norms and reliable standards for specific ages in later life, either in behavior or in bodily function. Therefore, it is wrong, and perhaps dangerous, to state that high blood pressure, early memory loss, or digestive and urinary tract problems in an individual are "normal for her/his age". This can result in failure to diagnose and treat the condition or to take the person's symptoms seriously. Alternatively, the normal processes of ageing are often interpreted as symptoms of treatable disease. As a result, medications are prescribed without clear indications leading to polypharmacy and excessive drug usage. The distinction between normal ageing and pathology is drawn clearly and the relevance of that distinction to the clinical assessment, diagnosis, and management of patients, particularly the prescription of medication, is well emphasized. Clear protocols for the prescription of many psychotropic drugs are also presented.

Five psychiatric conditions—depression, dementia, delirium, paranoid disorders and substance (alcohol and drug) abuse—are described in separate chapters. The authors note the paramount importance of accurate diagnosis. An inaccurate diagnosis can result in wrong treatment, failure to identify a potentially curable disease, and perhaps death of the patient. In the geriatric population, diagnostic accuracy often requires the highest skills of the physician and advice from a consultant internist, neurologist, or psychiatrist. Delirium is usually acute and is most commonly caused by toxicity from infection or drugs, or from withdrawal. In many cases it is curable if appropriate action is taken. If not, the outcome may be rapid fatality. High diagnostic skill may be required to differentiate depression from dementia but often the correct diagnosis is missed because both alternatives are not considered. Similarly, there can be difficulty in correctly diagnosing paranoid symptoms in the elderly. The following clinical illustration is relatively common: A severely withdrawn patient, transferred to a geriatric assessment unit after two years in a nursing home, seemed to be more aware of the environment than one would expect in someone severely demented. After a complete clinical assessment, the patient responded dramatically to appropriate treatment for depression.

The enthusiasm for accurate diagnosis often wanes in cases where there is no clear-cut clinical picture, no specific treatment and where the outcome is not a cure but chronic disease and variable disability. Physicians sometimes tend to lose interest in patients where diagnosis is difficult and treatment is diffuse. Yet it is precisely for such patients that the multi-disciplinary team can provide treatment and management of great benefit. While a precise diagnostic label may be elusive, a clear identification of each problem facing the patient and family is vital. Often each patient's problems are unique, depending on the physical and mental status, the personality and remaining assets, and the social support network. When each problem is clearly stated and the plan of management agreed upon and written down, it is more likely that care will be consistent and evaluation of outcome becomes possible. Even when a diagnosis has already been made, this problem-oriented approach makes sense to patients and families since diagnostic labels may be confusing and frightening. In addition, when the many small components of a patient's disabilities are identified and dealt with, the general status may be greatly improved. *Psycho-geriatrics: A Practical Handbook* provides countless suggestions for the resolution or palliation of many disabilities of the elderly with mental disorders.

Assessment of the older person is often difficult because of the complexity of the disease picture, often involving a mixture of mental, physical, and social problems. The first step must be to interview the patient to ensure that s/he does not feel s/he is being ignored or that decisions are being made without her/his knowledge. Even if full information is not obtainable due to impaired mental function, the clinical interview may at least identify significant emotional disorders and cognitive impairments. Information from the family or other informants is useful for corroboration and for understanding the relationship of the problems to the social setting in which the patient is embedded. One of the major thrusts and strengths of this book lies in its emphasis on and clear descriptions of the clinical assessment process, including examples of specific questions to elicit various symptoms.

The behavior of elderly patients may be "difficult" in the sense that it is inappropriate, may occur unexpectedly, and may be dangerous for the patient and/or other people. Correct management is dependent upon a correct diagnosis if it is a new phenomenon. More commonly, such behavior is episodic and recurrent in someone whose underlying condition has already been diagnosed correctly. Successful management of difficult behavior depends on understanding the psychological and social dynamics, and the patient's perspective. Whether the choice is to use medications, adopt a different care plan or modify the environment, or a mix of these, will depend on understanding this complex picture and on having the resources to respond.

Whether we are health care professionals, administrators, or program planners, we too often underestimate the problems a family must face when an elderly member requires ongoing care. In spite of contrary evidence, the family is still, and probably will continue to be, the greatest resource and asset for the care and protection of the very old or disabled person. However, we must appreciate not only the kinds of care families provide but also the social cost to individuals in doing so. Community support services and respite care can help the family caregivers, but we know that even permanent institutional care does not alleviate the family's concern and stress. Professionals and families should know how community resources can be tapped. Unfortunately, in many communities, support services are limited, and the major expansion of such services that is required is given a lower priority by government than hospital services. The various roles performed by family and other community-based caregivers is well described in this informative book.

The ageing of the population is inevitable. Whether the increased longevity is seen as an addition of healthy, active years, or as a burden, will depend on whether or not our society accepts seniors as participants and valued contributors. Prevention and improved treatment of many of the diseases of later life may be possible through research, thus enabling the population not only to live longer but also to enjoy a healthy, active old age. Even those with disabilities may enjoy better health if we carefully diagnose and treat the underlying conditions and provide more supportive environments. This book provides useful and practical information for all practitioners dealing with elderly people and enables them to help their patients with confidence.

J. Ronald D. Bayne M.D., F.R.C.P.(C), F.A.C.P.
Professor of Medicine (gerontology)
McMaster University
President, Canadian Association on Gerontology
Chairman, Gerontology Research Council of Ontario

Contents

Preface and Acknowledgments

All the world's a stage, and all the men and women merely players:
They have their exits and their entrances; And one man in his
time plays many parts, his acts being seven ages ... Last scene
of all, that ends this strange eventful history, is second childishness
and mere oblivion, sans teeth, sans eyes, sans taste, sans everything.

Act II, Scene VII
As You Like It
Shakespeare

The purpose of this book is to present information about mental disorder
in later life. The book is addressed to those health care professionals with
various backgrounds working in psychiatry, geriatrics, gerontology and other
related fields. This requires that the content be comprehensive, practical, and
relevant to provide a full description of the scope of psychogeriatrics. Such
an approach must take into consideration the differing needs of professionals
working in acute care hospitals, in palliative care units, in long-term care and
residential facilities, and in the community. In addition, the different professional
backgrounds—approaches to clinical management and responsibilities of nurses,
physicians, occupational therapists, physiotherapists, social workers and others—
must be acknowledged. Therefore, the various chapters of this handbook provide
very concise and practical information and management protocols for the practice
of psychogeriatrics by all of those disciplines in the above-noted clinical settings.

The book arose directly from the clinical experience of the authors, all
of whom are present or former members of the staff of the Community
Psychogeriatric Service in Metropolitan Toronto. It is the goal of this service
to provide consultative, educational, and co-ordinating services to caregivers
working with the elderly. In pursuit of this goal, we have acquired an extensive
working knowledge of the needs of many professionals both to understand
and to manage emotional disorder in their patients. Over the years we have
developed and refined a series of educational seminars on psychogeriatrics
which were attended by large numbers of health professionals and others. They
have identified the information that is most helpful and necessary to solve the
problems encountered in the course of daily clinical practice. This book has
been written in response to their demand for a permanent record of this
educational material and the contents represent a distillation of our thoughts
about what is most important.

As alluded to throughout the book, the most appropriate paradigm or unifying concept for both the normal and pathological sequelae of ageing is that of "loss". The net effect of ageing, in varying degrees, is an accumulation of physical and psychological losses. There is a progressive decline in physical integrity through normal wear and tear, the acquisition of chronic or degenerative diseases, and often an increased susceptibility to acute illness. The psychological losses encountered when growing old are protean. They may be brought about by changes in social roles and by the geographic separation from and deaths of relatives and friends.

Thus, it is not difficult to appreciate that Shakespeare's grim description of life's last scene may be regarded as the normal and natural outcome of ageing. Unfortunately, this description has too often become a stereotype for the aged—infirm of body and mind, irrelevant and non-contributory to society. However, the vast majority of the elderly population (defined arbitrarily as those over 65 years) do not fit this picture. They accumulate the above-noted losses but they remain very functional and they do contribute as valued members of society. Therefore, an attempt has been made to place the field of psychogeriatrics in the context of the processes which occur with normal ageing.

The first section of the book describes the various biological, psychological, and sociological changes which occur with ageing. Some of the most common mental disorders presenting in the geriatric population are described in the second section of the book. A description of the assessment of patients and specific aspects of the management of mental disorders and behavioral problems are presented in the third section, and in the fourth section the contributions of family and community resources to the maintenance of the elderly in the community are described.

The authors would like to express appreciation to a number of institutions, organizations and individuals who have contributed to the development and continuing operation of the Community Psychogeriatric Service and/or to the production of this book: The Alzheimer Society (Metropolitan Toronto Branch) for a grant to assist in the preparation of the manuscript; the Ontario Ministry of Health for funding the Community Psychogeriatric Service; Ms. K. Austin, co-ordinating editor, and Ms. S. Gilchrist, publishing director, Gage Educational Publishing Company, for their editorial assistance; and, Mrs. J. Miklossy and Ms. M. Chuso for typing successive drafts of the manuscript. His co-authors also wish to express appreciation to Dr. B. Martin for his special contribution. His enthusiasm, constructive criticism, and encouragement were vital factors in the accomplishment of this endeavor.

Part One
AGEING

1

Normal Ageing

Deborah M. Clark, B.S.W., C.S.W., M.Ed.
and Lynda A. Perry, M.S.W., C.S.W.

This chapter presents an overview of the biological, psychological, and sociological changes that are considered to be normal accompaniments of ageing. Based on the 1981 census, 9.7 percent of the Canadian population is age 65 and over. This age group is expected to include approximately 13 percent of the population by the end of the century and almost 20 percent by the year 2031. Bearing these statistics in mind, the overall need for health and social services for the elderly will expand markedly. Therefore, health professionals need to become more knowledgeable about the normal ageing process in order to address effectively the somewhat unique problems presented by older persons and their families.

An understanding of what constitutes normal ageing is essential before one can recognize pathology. Some of the biological theories of ageing and the physical changes which occur in body tissues are described. The section on psychological aspects summarizes developmental tasks of old age, changes in personality, interpersonal relationships, and cognitive functioning. The sociological factors of status and power, role expectations, and economics which may affect the health of the elderly and the provision of services are also considered.

BIOLOGICAL CHANGES WITH AGEING

Life expectancy is the average number of years of life remaining for an individual at a given age. Based on the 1981 census, the average life expectancy in Canada for newborn males is 71.5 and for newborn females is 78.7. This has been slowly increasing as the result of improved medical care. Life expectancy may be influenced by sex, standard of living, and lifestyle factors (for example, diet, stress, and substance abuse), with women living longer in most countries.

Individuals in a specific age group may die earlier or live longer consistent with their unique genetic and family history, disease development, and absence or presence of mental disorders. Quite apart from these unique or individual factors, there are biological changes that occur in all individuals as part of normal ageing.

Biological or physical ageing consists of the progressive decline or loss of physiological capacities and functions. The changes that occur are normal for all persons, although they may take place at different rates and depend upon accompanying circumstances in the individual's life. Many changes in body structure and function are lifelong processes that begin to take on significance in the fifth and sixth decade. As ageing occurs, there is increasing vulnerability to degenerative disease such as arthritis and coronary arteriosclerosis. In terms of physical changes, normal ageing begins at approximately 30 years of age, after which most physiologic functions decline at a slow rate.

It is extremely important to be aware of and to recognize age-related changes as being distinct from disease. If a change due to normal ageing is misidentified as a disease process, a treatment may be applied that was never intended to reverse the ageing process. The more aggressive the intervention, the greater the potential for iatrogenic harm. Conversely, if a disease process is attributed to normal ageing, treatment of the medical condition may be neglected. To complicate things further, old people are often reluctant to report illness because they are instilled with the same ageism that affects the rest of society—normal ageing processes are regarded as synonymous with disease. [In fact, the age of onset and/or clinical presentation and course of some diseases are unique to the elderly.] These illnesses may be conceptualized in two groups. Some occur in persons of any age but present differently in the elderly (for example, thyroid disease, myocardial infarction, carcinoma, and depression). The other group includes those diseases more prevalent in old age (for example, temporal arteritis, polymyalgia rheumatica, herpes zoster/shingles, and, Parkinson's disease).

Biological Theories of Ageing

Theories of ageing must explain the fundamental nature and mechanisms of the ageing process, and its manifestations and effects on bodily functions. Biological theories are concerned with cellular changes that give rise to metabolic deficiencies as a result of slow repair processes, chromosomal alterations, or accumulation of waste products. Cell division continues to shape the human organism throughout the life span. Among the many theories of ageing, the following are summarized: free radical, cross linkage, immunologic, somatic mutation and error, wear and tear, stress adaptation, and single organ theories. It should be noted that they are not mutually exclusive but tend to complement one another.

Non-genetic Theories

These theories presume that time-related changes in molecules and other structural elements of the cells impair their effectiveness.

Wear and Tear Theory

It is assumed that the body behaves like a machine and, thus, with repeated use, parts wear out and the machinery ultimately comes to a halt. This theory suggests that human beings are only made to last 100 years or so.

Free Radical Theory

Free radicals are chemicals whose outer orbit contains an unpaired electron which makes these substances highly reactive. It is hypothesized that free radicals contribute to age changes by combining with essential molecules, that is, the free radicals attach themselves to other molecules damaging or altering their original structure or function over the course of a lifetime. Free radical damage to protein or deoxyribonucleic acid (DNA) theoretically could produce profound effects and lead to cross linkages (see Cross Linkage Theory). It is not known whether free radical production is a fundamental cause of ageing or if it is an associated effect.

Cross Linkage Theory (also called Collagen Theory)

This theory applies mostly to non-cellular material, especially collagen, which constitutes 25 percent of total body protein. High concentrations of collagen appear in skin, tendons, bone, muscle, blood vessels, and the heart. This theory suggests that chemical reactions create strong bonds between molecular structures that are normally separate. Thus, the formation of these cross linkages alters the physical and chemical properties of molecules involved so that they no longer function in the same manner. A formation of cross links results in the well-known age-associated changes in the skin. While the accumulation of cross link molecules may be a primary cause of ageing, there is no convincing evidence that these changes represent the ultimate cause of ageing.

Genetic Theories

Genetic theories of ageing are based on the assumption that the life span is determined by information contained in the DNA molecules of the genes. Ageing might be attributed to an underlying series of orderly programmed genetic events that shut down or slow down essential physiological phenomena. While the genetic program may set upper limits of life span, other factors such as gender, heredity, nutrition as well as psychosocial influences play a major role in determining life span.

Somatic Mutation Theory

According to this theory, progressive accumulation of mutations or other generalized damage in DNA leads to incapacitation of individual cells. This theory suggests that exposure to radiation accelerates the ageing process.

Error Theory

This theory expands upon the somatic theory to include cumulative errors in ribonucleic acid (RNA), protein, and enzyme synthesis. According to this theory, ageing and death of the cell are the result of errors which may occur at any point in the information transfer resulting in the formation of a protein or enzyme which is defective and, therefore is unable to function properly.

Physiological Theories

These theories focus on the interaction between cells and organs and attempt to explain ageing on the basis of impaired performance of a single organ or of a physiological control mechanism.

Single Organ Theories

Ageing results in the progressive deterioration of blood vessels due to atherosclerosis. Alternatively, ageing is due to the slowing down of the metabolic processes caused by thyroid failure. These theories have been criticized because the observed changes may simply be the result of more fundamental causes, for example, genetic programming.

Stress Adaptation Theory

Ageing may result from the cumulative effects of life stresses, leaving a residual impairment from which an individual does not completely recover. However, this assumption of long-term damage is not supported by experimental data.

Immunologic Theories

The immune system protects the body against invading micro-organisms and mutant cells which may develop in the body. According to the immunologic theories, the fundamental impairment may be a declining ability to recognize slight deviations in molecular structure or cell characteristics so that mutant cells that would ordinarily be eliminated are no longer recognized and are permitted to grow.

Physical Changes in Body Systems

The major results of ageing may be a breakdown of regulatory mechanisms, primarily those involving the endocrine, neurological, and immune systems. The pattern of age decrement is individualized and the rate of decline varies from one function to another and from one individual to another. There is no simple cause and effect relationship between the degree of structural impairment and the presence of impaired function or manifest disease. A hallmark of health is the ability to maintain a steady state; however, with advancing age, capacity for homeostasis gradually declines. The range of adjustment and adaptation becomes smaller and narrower. The ensuing sections review age related changes in body tissues and function which one would expect to find with advancing years.

Skin and Tissue Elasticity

The aged skin loses resilience and moisture, taking on a characteristic dryness (meaning roughness), and resulting in wrinkling. Age related changes in hair color, density, and distribution are also widely recognized. Sun exposure increases skin tissue changes. Elasticity affects blood vessel integrity, particularly that of the arteries. There is little flow change to the arteries in the brain but perfusion of the liver and the kidneys shows significant changes in the amount of blood brought to these organs. Calcification of the arterial system is a linear function of age. Lung elasticity declines and is a contributing factor to a decrease in oxygen capacity.

Cardiovascular System

The heart size remains unchanged in the absence of cardiovascular disease. The rate at which blood is pumped through the heart and the maximum amount of air that can be pumped in and out of the lungs declines at a rate of approximately one percent per year. Reduced efficiency of the heart muscle and contractile strength are reflected in a smaller cardiac output. Under non-stressful conditions, smaller output is adequate for the average person to function; however, diminished cardiac output becomes significant when the aged individual is stressed physically or mentally by illness and/or activity. With age, there is an increase in the time required for the heart rate to return to the normal level once it is elevated. Ageing increases blood pressure by stiffening blood vessels and increasing peripheral resistance. Blood pressure, systolic more than diastolic, increases with age for both men and women.

Respiratory System

Changes in lung performance are not obvious but with exertion or stress, dyspnea may appear. The lungs do not shrink in size but become more rigid. Total lung capacity is not significantly altered but rather it is redistributed. The cough reflex is frequently depressed.

Fat Tissue

Of all body tissue, the fatty layer fluctuates the most throughout life and is subject to greater change. Fat tissue has a major role in the body's adjustment to temperature change. With the loss of fat tissue, the body's natural insulation is lost. In addition, the sweat glands decrease in size, number, and activity causing a decline in the efficiency of the body's cooling system which can result in an increased risk of heat exhaustion and hypothermia.

Endocrine System

The aged exhibit a decreased ability to metabolize glucose. The pancreas fails to produce sufficient insulin in the presence of blood glucose, either as a result of reduced peripheral sensitivity of the pancreas or as a consequence of declining insulin response. Age-related glucose intolerance may be confused with diabetes and perhaps lead to unnecessary treatment. Decrease in thyroid activity is apparent in the slowing of the metabolic rate and oxygen utilization of the body. Women may experience changes due to a decrease in estrogen secretions following menopause. Diminished hormone levels lead to atrophy of the ovaries, uterus and vaginal tissue. Ageing men develop firmer testes and a tendency for prostatic hypertrophy, which is benign in most cases.

Bone and Muscle

Osteoporosis, due to progressive bone loss, is a major problem in women after menopause. This condition is much more common in women than in men, in the elderly than in the young, and in whites than in blacks. Vitamin D and calcium and adequate physical activity are important in building and maintaining a larger bone mass. Generally with age, bones become porous and brittle with an increased risk of fractures which take longer to mend. The spine may assume a characteristic curve known as kyphosis. The development of kyphosis and osteoporosis are two factors that contribute to the shorter stature of the aged. Individuals who exercise regularly do not lose as much bone and muscle mass or tone as those who remain sedentary. Muscle strength decreases in proportion to the decrease in muscle mass. General physical strength also declines markedly.

Gastrointestinal System

The digestive system handles age-related changes better than most systems in the body. With normal ageing, oesophageal motility declines somewhat. Dentition is an important adjunct to the gastrointestinal system and any substantial loss may affect digestive activity. There is a decrease in salivary secretions which can impair further the ability to chew food. Vitamin and mineral deficiencies may result from faulty absorption and inadequate diet. Many gastrointestinal problems that present with advancing age are functional; that is, there is no physical cause that can be detected.

The internal sphincter of the large intestine loses its muscle tone and can create problems with bowel evacuation. The problems of constipation and the use and abuse of laxatives in the elderly may require nursing and/or medical attention.

Urinary Tract

With advancing age, ureter, bladder and urethra have decreased muscle tone. The volume capacity of the bladder decreases. As a result, many healthy aged experience frequency and urgency to urinate.

Creatinine clearance is markedly decreased as a result of the decline in renal function. There is impaired renal clearance of drugs resulting in drug accumulation; hence the high risk of drug toxicity in the elderly. (See also Chapter 11.)

Sensory Systems

All five senses gradually lose their acuity with old age. Taste sensations with old age diminish due to loss of taste bud receptors. The major flavors of sour, bitter, sweet, and salty are less clearly discriminated. Sense of smell diminishes in proportion to taste. There is also a decreased response to pain. The lowering of normal pain signals may create potentially dangerous situations in the aged. Serious diseases (for example, myocardial infarction and appendicitis) may present with less acute pain than in younger patients, and, as a result, medical attention may be delayed.

There are several specific age-related changes in vision. Deterioration may be attributable to natural changes such as retinal loss, decreased pupil diameter, lens opacities, loss of lens elasticity and to vascular, metabolic, or endocrine problems. There is a decreased ability to see at a distance after age 50. The pupil size becomes smaller affecting the amount of light that reaches the retina. There is also reduced ability to re-focus at varying distances. Due to the reduced amount of light reaching the retina there is a decreased ability to adapt to the dark.

The efficiency of pupillary constriction and dilation compromises the ability to adapt vision to dim light and darkness. There is a decrease in color perception (blues, violets and greens). This is why, for example, staff in a long-term care facility should wear yellow name badges.

Age associated changes in vision, also known as presbyopia, occur between the ages of 45 and 55. Partial or complete loss of presbyopic sight may occur in several ways. Senile macular degeneration, caused by hardening and obstruction of the retinal arteries, may cause the loss of central vision but peripheral vision remains intact. Glaucoma, resulting from increased pressure within the eye, may damage and eventually destroy the retina. The lens of the eye may become opaque as cataracts develop. Vision is reduced because light cannot pass through.

Auditory changes occur gradually. Loss of hearing is a common occurrence of old age. Decrements in hearing acuity, speech intelligibility, and discrimination of pitch (especially in speech frequencies), are referred to as presbycusis. Sounds tend to fuse and distinctions between background noise and conversation are difficult. The ability to hear is a major avenue of communication. Significant hearing loss is not only frustrating to the individual but is threatening to self-esteem. Hearing loss involves social consequences and one may see a vicious circle of less participation and socialization leading to isolation and suspiciousness that can progress to paranoia.

Altered proprioception or the sense of the body's position in space can lead to considerable difficulties in balance and spatial orientation.

Brain

The most readily recognizable feature of the aged central nervous system is a decreased brain weight. The weight of the brain declines approximately 10 to 15 percent by age 70 from that of young adulthood. The loss of cells is not uniform throughout the brain—the neurons of the cerebral cortex are most vulnerable. While the loss of brain cells begins in the third or fourth decade and continues steadily thereafter, functional ability may not be significantly affected as a result of the compensatory activity of remaining cells.

Intelligence and Learning

In the absence of organic brain disease, an individual's intellectual abilities remain relatively stable into late life. There is little decline in verbal intelligence with age but performance on psychomotor tasks shows significant decline. Older people are typically more concerned with accuracy and consistency than speed. (The relationship between ageing and intelligence is also discussed in Chapter 5.)

With age, there is a slowing in thought processes rather than an absolute loss of intellectual capacity. Older individuals frequently compensate for these age associated changes with increased general knowledge and problem solving abilities. Although old people usually take longer to learn something new it is not impossible for them to learn new information. The learning process of the older adult is discussed later in this chapter. It should be remembered that individual differences in level of intellectual functioning are maintained into old age. Major cognitive loss is always due to disease and warrants medical investigation.

Memory Loss

While healthy and active elderly people may complain of forgetting names and dates, this form of forgetfulness is typically benign in nature. Benign memory loss associated with normal ageing is generally the loss of unimportant details or parts of an experience that occurred in the remote past. What is forgotten on one occasion may be easily recalled at a later time. Usually, the older person is aware of this failure in recall and makes appropriate compensations. In contrast, malignant memory loss in an older person involves a marked inability to recall events of the recent past (including not only the insignificant details but the experience itself). This form of memory loss may be accompanied by disorientation and confabulation. Establishing routines, simplifying tasks to be performed, and use of repetition may be effective management strategies with a person with declining memory functioning. Refer to Chapters 5 and 9 for further description of types and assessment of memory loss.

The sleep/wake cycle is influenced by the brain. In general, the aged do require less sleep. The aged person experiences less rapid eye movement episodes (REM) and deep sleep than in earlier life. (See also Chapter 11.)

Sexual Function

Interest and capacity to enjoy sexual relationships continues throughout the life span. The ability to have sexual relations will depend upon a number of factors, including the availability of a partner (this may be a problem with women outliving men), health status (both physical and mental), and privacy.

There are physiological changes that take place with ageing and their effect on sexual functioning is outlined in Table 1.1.

TABLE 1.1

Changes in Sexual Function with Age

Men

a. Erection may become less hard.
b. Ability to postpone ejaculation for a longer period of time usually increases.
c. It may take longer to achieve an erection and reach orgasm.
d. Orgasm may be less intense and release less forceful.
e. It may take longer before a second erection is possible.

Women

Many of the physical changes in women result from lowered hormone levels and these changes may include:

a. A thinning of the vaginal walls which can cause irritation during intercourse.
b. With ageing a woman typically requires more time to achieve vaginal lubrication.
c. Contractions experienced during orgasm sometimes become uncomfortable.
d. A longer time may be needed to become aroused.
e. Orgasm may be less intense.

These changes may affect some people and not others. They may take place at different ages for different individuals and may show up in varying degrees. Sexual performance in both sexes may be affected by certain medications (i.e. tranquillizers, antihypertensives, and alcohol). Diabetes, anemia, and other physical disorders can interfere with sexual function, as can physical and emotional stress.

PSYCHOLOGICAL ASPECTS OF AGEING

This discussion of the psychology of late life includes the developmental tasks of ageing, personality factors, interpersonal relationships, and cognitive functioning. (See also Chapter 3.)

Developmental Tasks

The notion that the elderly still have developmental tasks to perform may seem contradictory and has been frequently overlooked. However, development is a lifelong process and there are specific tasks appropriate to later years. The major developmental task of old age is "to resolve one's life conflicts successfully, to review and integrate one's past events with a personal value system which reflects the achievement of life's satisfaction, the emergence of a developed life philosophy, and the acquisition of wisdom" (Birren & Renner 1981, 249).

Erik Erickson (1950) has described eight developmental tasks from infancy through to old age. Associated with these stages are eight major crises which each person must face and resolve in order to progress to the next. The fundamental task of old age is to attain "ego integrity". An ageing individual should appreciate that s/he is nearing death and accept, understand, and value life as it has been lived. Failure to achieve integrity may lead to despair.

Successfully achieving a sense of personal integrity in old age depends on having succeeded in earlier tasks such as becoming productive, intimate, and creative.

The process by which an older person achieves such integration is a matter of some dispute. For example, some theorists suggest that as people age they increasingly become inwardly focussed, making a smaller emotional investment in people and places. This process focusses on the person slowly disengaging from the world as s/he comes to terms with her/himself. Others find that people who remain busy and socially involved are more likely to age successfully. These concepts need not be mutually exclusive. A person may wish to retain some activities and yet lead a quieter life with some time for reflection. Different patterns will be more or less successful for different people.

In general, the developmental tasks of old age involve coming to terms with oneself as a person and as a member of society. It is important when working with the elderly to support this process. Listening with genuine interest to reminiscences and acknowledging the strengths and achievements involved in past activities is one important way to assist an older person to think positively of his or her self-worth. Seeking advice about matters within the person's expertise is another very concrete way of indicating that a person's contribution is valued. Of course, older people who remain active will find many opportunities to enhance their positive sense of themselves.

Personality Changes

In considering personality factors in old age it is important to realize that there is no particular personality pattern typical of older people. In fact, older people may tend to be more unique than younger people. They are the product of many years of both unique and shared experiences.

The question of whether a personality changes with age has not been definitively answered. Many studies indicate that personality tends to be rather stable over a lifetime and that in fact people become more like themselves as they age. Other studies, both cross-sectional and longitudinal, have found changes in personality traits as people age. These changes are attributed to underlying needs unmet earlier in life, changed social situations, changed expectations, or changes in role status. For example, a woman who spent all her life nurturing a family, may in her later years decide to pursue the education she always felt she lacked. Involvement in her new occupation may result in profound behavioral changes such as neglect of family and home. Yet viewed from another perspective these profound changes may be merely a new form of expression for a woman who had always focussed her energy single-mindedly towards a creative task.

An example of how a change in normative expectations may alter a personality is seen in the person who has believed the myth that productivity stops at age 65. This person may retire from 45 or 50 years of paid employment with the expectation that one's role in life is now simply one of continuous relaxation with no expectation to do anything productive. S/he may soon become bored, listless, and irritable from lack of challenge and stimulation.

Numerous studies have attempted to identify personality traits common to the elderly or to challenge stereotypes about older people. These studies have found that older people's morale and life satisfaction are as high as that of younger people. They are not socially isolated and lonely. They are not always irritated or angry. They remain interested in sexual relations and social activities. Marriages surviving into later years often provide a high level of satisfaction for the couple involved. (See also Chapter 14).

Interpersonal Relationships

Relationships with others is another important aspect of the psychology of ageing. Many factors affect the number and quality of interpersonal relationships of older people including occupational, marital and health status, family dynamics, and environment. Most older people are retired and as a result lose ready access to colleagues and co-workers. Some of these relationships may be maintained socially, but many will end immediately or shortly after retirement. Many people re-invest the time no longer spent in employment by expanding their social activities and relationships. Others become more socially isolated and withdrawn when work no longer provides a forum for their social needs. Still others replace work with a second career or with volunteer positions which can contribute not only to their social relationships but also to their sense of productivity and self-esteem.

The older person who has had a lifetime of satisfying relationships will likely find ways to continue the old and to form new relationships throughout the later years. However, sometimes even outgoing and friendly people find themselves without meaningful relationships in later years. Circumstances such as a person's ill-health or that of a spouse may decrease and eventually eliminate social contact. It is very important to assist a person in this situation to develop and maintain social contacts as a way of restoring the quality of their lives. For example, one 75 year old gentleman whose wife was suffering from a dementia which required constant supervision found that he could maintain important relationships through becoming a ham radio operator. He was able to maintain contact with a wide range of people and stimulate his mind, while still being alert to his wife's needs.

Older people retain the same needs as younger people for love and affection and respect. Meeting these needs becomes more difficult in later years in a society which defines older people as unappealing and uninteresting. A vicious circle may be developed wherein an older person lacking in close relationships reaches out for affection. The advance may be viewed as repulsive by the recipient and the older person is labelled as demanding or intrusive. Further isolation may result in decreased opportunity to meet the legitimate need for affection.

Cognitive Functioning

Intellectual or cognitive functioning does show some change with age. While early studies found a significant decrease in intellectual function as people aged, these findings were affected by methodological problems. In these studies, young people who were accustomed to test-taking performed best. Performance appeared to deteriorate progressively from the 20 year old group to the oldest group. More recent, longitudinal studies which compare the performance of the same group of people at periodic intervals, find stability in intellectual functioning into the eighth decade. (The relationship between ageing and cognitive function is also discussed earlier in this chapter and in Chapter 5.)

Some general conclusions about the relationship between age and intellectual or cognitive function are: at age 50, speed of thinking and reading tends to decline; at age 55, social deprivation may lead to decline in ability; between ages 60 to 75, some decline in some abilities is seen in *some* people; and over age 85, some decline in some abilities is seen in *most* people.

Some cognitive abilities are more "age-resistant" than others. Among the abilities which tend not to decrease with advancing age are those which involve "crystalized functions". Older people are quite adept at learning new information when it can be related to a well-established knowledge base. Some of the cognitive abilities which involve this type of associative mental function are general knowledge, practical judgment, and dexterity. Less age-resistant abilities are those which rely on "fluid functions". Mental agility, concentration, and memory are examples of abilities which are more likely to decline with age.

Older people are able to learn new information and skills provided adequate time and practice is allowed. They are more concerned with accuracy and consistency than speed.

When trying to teach an older person something new the following teaching principles are important. Link the new skill or information to something already familiar and ensure that the person understands the purpose of the teaching. This will yield better results than trying to teach material which appears to be irrelevant. Also, presenting material in a logical sequence makes it easier to assimilate. Because the older brain works a little slower, it is important to pace teaching to ensure that the older person grasps each concept or task before moving on to the next step. Repetition over a period of time until the new skill or information has been fully integrated is a helpful teaching strategy.

SOCIOLOGICAL CHANGES WITH AGEING

Social Status and Power

Status refers to an individual's or group's position on the power hierarchy of society. The higher one's status, the more one is recognized as having power. Power involves the ability to obtain one's objectives and to influence others in order to serve one's own interests. Power and status are not absolutes. A person may have a great deal of status and power within one's own family group and yet have a very low status in society in general. The opposite can also be true.

A number of factors influence the position held by seniors within a society. One such factor is the stability of the society. Seniors tend to lose status in rapidly changing societies where their life experience is viewed as irrelevant or no longer valid. Another factor involves the proportion of older people in the society. Where there are fewer elderly, their scarcity tends to make them more valued. A third factor involves the extent to which older people are engaged in activities which are considered to be useful or productive—the greater the perceived productivity, the higher the status.

These three factors are discussed briefly as they pertain to North American society. If these factors are valid considerations in ascribing status, it is not difficult to see that being old is not a high status position within our society and that there are strong pressures towards an even lower status for tomorrow's elderly. Society is changing rapidly. Social structures and mores are evolving almost as rapidly as technology is advancing. For example, the typical family structure has evolved from a strong extended family through a mobile nuclear family to the single adult with or without children in the space of less than 50 years. These rapid changes contribute to people discounting as obsolete the wisdom which the older generation has achieved through life experience.

The second factor is also true. To be old in our society is no longer rare and is becoming more common. In 1981, there were twice as many people age 75 and over in Ontario alone as there had been in all of Canada in 1931. This trend is expected to continue. The oldest age group, those aged 85 and over, is the most rapidly growing segment of our society.

Performance of useful activities, the third factor cited as influencing status, is one which has some potential for improving the status of the elderly. Senior citizens are becoming more vocal about their value to society. They are rejecting the notion that life after 65 should be for passive leisure and are seeking new challenges in education, second careers, and volunteerism. The marketplace is beginning to recognize the consuming potential of this rapidly growing group and are offering products and services tailored to their needs and wants.

For those few elderly who do fit the stereotype of being poor, sickly, and slow, status and power are very minimal. To the extent that a person is dependent on others for basic needs, that person loses status and power. The resulting low expectations lead to caregivers allowing the dependent elderly few opportunities to use and enhance their remaining abilities. Thus a vicious circle develops in which skills diminish, self-esteem is lowered, and dependency is increased, confirming the societal attitude that the elderly are incompetent. Therefore, those caring for the dependent elderly must be particularly vigilant to accord status to the frail elderly to minimize the dependency that may be created and to enhance their quality of life. There must be an awareness of ageism and its deleterious effects in order to combat it. Normal ageing is neither least ageing nor debility but a life stage with problems to be resolved and challenges to be met.

Stress and Changing Roles

Any change which poses a threat to a person's life, status, relationships, possessions, or belief system will cause a stress reaction in the individual. Much of the research on stress has focussed on the impact of major life events on health. Many studies have found that people experiencing a number of major changes within a short time period are likely to suffer ill-health as a consequence.

While recent research questions the methodology of earlier studies, it is likely that there is some relationship between stressful events and health status. Current research is considering the subjective evaluation of the event to be a factor in the amount of stress associated with a change. The elderly generally define life events as being less stress producing than do younger adults. This does not minimize the importance of stress for the elderly because it appears that even small amounts of stress can result in marked impact on the health of an older person.

The later years bring with them many changes which threaten the individual's lifestyle. Many of these changes involve loss. Loss of employment through retirement, loss of companionship through death, loss of social life through ill-health of self or others, and loss of familiar surroundings through relocation to a lower maintenance setting are all potential stressors for the elderly. Other changes involve new opportunities. The birth of grandchildren and increased time to pursue interests are examples of changes which may be viewed positively and yet still create stress.

Over a lifetime, individuals learn to cope with varying levels of stress. This learning is facilitated by stress which occurs at a slow enough rate so as not to overwhelm. The increased rate of change with age may tax the ability of the person to deal with stress. In addition, the older person may well have fewer resources to aid her/him in coping with stressful events. One prominent stress researcher, Hans Selye (1974), suggests that each person has a finite amount of "adaptation energy" available for a lifetime. This would suggest that an older person is likely to have smaller reserves of "adaptation energy" available. An older person is also likely to have fewer coping mechanisms available.

Economic Changes

The economics of ageing is relevant at both the personal and societal level. On a personal level, with Old Age Assistance and Guaranteed Income Supplement, seniors need not be destitute, but unless low rental housing can be procured, they will have difficulty providing themselves with more than minimal essentials. While some costs go down with advancing age (i.e. food and clothing) other new costs are incurred and health and drug costs may rise. Many senior citizens have a very strong aversion to accepting government assistance even when they are entitled to financial, recreational, and other services.

The reality is that in Canada nearly half of the elderly rely on government allowances for their total income and only 13 percent have more than a minimal income from private pensions and investments. The average income of the elderly in Canada in 1978 was less than half the national average income. This reliance on government pensions which provide poverty level incomes is likely to continue. Less than half of employed Canadians have employer sponsored pensions and less than half of those provide survivors benefits. Older women who live longer and who have traditionally not participated in the workforce, are most likely to have incomes at or below the poverty line. This situation will improve slightly as more women are employed outside the home. However, women tend to work at low paying jobs and tend to drop out of the workforce during childbearing years, thus lowering their pension entitlements. Therefore, they will continue to be vulnerable to poverty in old age.

At the societal level of economics, there is much concern that the elderly are and will be a burden to the younger population. For example, statistics show that the elderly use twice as many medical services and almost four times the number of hospital-bed days than warranted by their proportion in the population. However, these figures can be misleading. Part of the problem is due not to the elderly but to the way in which our health delivery services are organized. More emphasis on the use of consultation from geriatricians and specialists in geriatric psychiatry could have two positive effects. Consultation is more cost effective than having everyone seen by specialists. Also, because specialists are scarce, more people can benefit from their expertise when they function as consultants in addition to their roles as clinicians. This larger impact benefits both patients and society through more accurate diagnosis and more effective treatment.

CONCLUSION

The health professional should be knowledgeable about the biological, sociological, and psychological changes associated with normal ageing in order to have a comprehensive understanding of the older person. This increased understanding will facilitate accurate assessment and formulation of appropriate interventions to help the elderly and their caregivers when abnormal ageing has been identified.

REFERENCES AND SUGGESTED READINGS

Besdine R. W. and K. L. Minaker. February 1983. "Aging: How Does It Affect Health?" *Patient Care.* 17: 21.

Birren J. E. and V. J. Renner. April 1981. "Concepts and Criteria of Mental Health and Aging." *American Journal of Orthopsychiatry.* 51.

Busse E. 1971. "Biologic and Sociologic Changes Affecting Adaptation In Mid and Later Life." *Annals In International Medicine.* 75: 115.

Cohen Leah. 1984. *Small Expectations—Society's Betrayal of Older Women.* Toronto: McClelland & Stewart.

Dowd J. J. 1980. *Stratification Among the Aged.* Monterey: Brooks/Cole Publishing Co.

Ebersole P. and P. Hess. 1981. *Toward Healthy Aging.* St. Louis: C. V. Mosby Co.

Erikson Erik. 1950. *Childhood and Society.* New York: W. W. Norton.

Goldstein S. and W. Reichel. 1978. "Physiological and Biological Aspects of Aging." *Clinical Aspects of Aging.* Baltimore: Williams & Wilkins Co.

Marshall V. 1980. *Aging in Canada: Social Perspectives.* Toronto: Fitzhenry & Whitside.

McPherson B. D. 1983. *Aging As A Social Process.* Toronto: Butterworths.

Palmore E. 1977. "Facts On Aging." *The Gerontologist.* 17: 315.

Renner V. J. and J. E. Birren. 1980. "Stress: Physiological and Psychological Mechanisms." *Handbook of Mental Health and Aging.* Englewood Cliffs: Prentice-Hall Inc.

Selye Hans. 1974. *Stress Without Distress.* New York: J. B. Lippincott.

Shock N. (ed.) 1962. *Biological Aspects of Aging.* New York: Columbia University Press.

Vanderzyl S. May/June 1979. "Psychosocial Theories of Aging: Activity Disengagement and Continuity." *Journal of Gerontological Nursing.* 5: 45.

Wasow M. and M. Loeb. 1977. "The Aged." *The Sexually Oppressed.* Ed. H. Gochras and J. S. Gochras. New York: Association Press.

Williamson J. B., A. Munley and L. Evans. 1980. *Aging In Society: An Introduction to Social Gerontology.* New York: Holt, Rinehart, & Winston.

2

Loss, Grief, and Adaptation

Mary K. Harrison, R.N., Ph.D.

Old age has been called a season of loss. Ageing individuals lose the role of working, contributing members of society and join children in the "dependency ratio" of society. Much of the western world does not recognize anyone who is not working as being of value. Decreases in income and declining health further enhance the perception of the elderly as dependents. As friends and relatives of similar age die or become ill, they constitute a reminder of what advancing years may bring. Caregivers who mean well may suggest moves to smaller living quarters or institutions which further compound the losses in ageing. Diminished energy and activity tolerance further remind the elderly of their body function losses. The rate and severity of chronic illness increases with age adding further losses. Because of the normal losses of ageing and illness-related losses, the elderly may be considered as being in a process of continual grief.

For other age groups, pathological grief is often the underlying cause of physical and mental problems. Research specific to the elderly is limited so that precise data about the incidence of pathological grief is only speculation. However, the amount of grief in an increasingly vulnerable population would suggest the potential for a high incidence. In addition, one might conceptualize that some of the emotional responses to chronic illness in the elderly are actually grief responses. Pathological grief reactions, true clinical depression or exacerbation of physical disease, can be outcomes of inadequate grief.

Understanding normal grief, facilitating its appropriate process, and enhancing coping and adaptation to chronic illness is an important intervention. Facilitating normal grieving in the elderly may prevent some of the complications mentioned and may enable both the elderly and their caregivers to maintain important and stimulating interaction. Enhancing coping and adaptation in chronic illness can assist in improving total functioning as well as improving life experience. In order to facilitate normal grieving effectively, there must be an understanding of normal grief, the special attributes of grief in the elderly, risk factors, and the facilitation process itself. That process can be accomplished with careful listening and empathic responses from the many professional and non-professional individuals who may already be in the elderly person's environment. It is not necessary to "pathologize" normal grief by introducing the psychiatric professional. However, changes in society have caused fewer individuals to look to religious leaders and institutions for help with grief. The emotional and physical responses that are part of normal grief can be very frightening; thus, the individual and non-psychiatric professional caregivers often seek out a mental health professional. Without some caution, this may paradoxically add to the burden of the elderly by labelling quite normal but disturbing symptoms of grief as being those of a mental illness.

Coping and adaptation to chronic illness involves a complex array of tasks and needs. Caregivers need to understand those tasks and the process of facilitating their accomplishment so that elderly individuals with chronic illness can live meaningful lives. A normal adaptive response is not a psychiatric illness and should not be so labelled to further inhibit performance.

DEFINITION OF GRIEF & TASKS OF MOURNING

Grief is the normal response to any loss, real or symbolic. Loss is experienced by the withdrawal of any meaningful relationship or role, change in physical functions, or loss of body part. Any change, whether positive or negative, planned or accidental, may be regarded as loss because each involves a letting go of some earlier relationship or self-system alteration. Again, it is important to emphasize that grief is normal. For a professional or a lay person, this is often difficult to comprehend because of the enormous emotional and often physical pain that characterizes normal grief.

Some of the emotional responses have been popularized. Indeed the linear emotional stages of the grief responses that have been so popularized may be an injustice to some people. Recent research indicates that stages of grief response are neither linear nor as time limited as initially indicated. A more appropriate way of looking at grief is to examine the function of the grief process for the human personality. The adaptation-to-loss model of the grief process parallels other developmental tasks of normal growth and development.

Four tasks have been identified:

1. To accept the reality of the loss
2. To emancipate emotionally from the ties with the deceased
3. To adjust to an environment without the deceased
4. To reinvest in a relationship as meaningful as the one that was lost

In examining these tasks it is apparent that each suggests both a variety of emotional responses and the means for its facilitation. For the individual to accept the reality of the loss, the loss must be experienced. In this process the individual experiences a variety of physical and emotional responses. Individuals who have experienced grief report somatic distress with waves of discomfort, for example, shortness of breath, a feeling of emptiness, changes in bowel and bladder habits, changes in appetite and sleep patterns as well as feelings of acute fear and anxiety. Often, identification with the illness behavior of the deceased is experienced with a resultant increased anxiety in the grieving individual. Cognitively, the grieving person is either preoccupied with or avoids thoughts of the deceased. Alternatively, the deceased may be idealized. This idealization further inhibits grieving the loss of the real person. The griever may show erratic judgment or impaired problem-solving ability. An individual often feels guilty and responsible for what happened. The griever berates her/himself for what s/he should have or could have done as well as what s/he did or did not do. Usual patterns of conduct may be lost with the individual's reactions. Warmth to others varies greatly often further inhibiting the support available. Impulsivity, both as an expression of poor judgment and of emotional distress, may interfere with the capacity to carry through on concrete tasks.

The tasks of accepting the reality of the loss and withdrawal from the emotional ties with the deceased continue to be accomplished as the griever experiences the loss and mourns the deceased. The initial response to loss is often a sense of disbelief and denial with the individual describing oneself as "going through the motions" or "frozen", but not really in touch with what has happened. When the individual does begin to deal with what has occurred, there is often crying, anger at being abandoned, and deep sadness. This sadness is often defined as depression but is not true clinical depression. It expresses itself in sporadic eating and sleeping problems, rapidly changing abilities to concentrate and follow through on activities and varying affective responses. The consistent symptoms over time that are the hallmark of a clinical depression are absent. (See also Chapter 4.)

The tasks of accepting the reality of the loss and the loosening of ties with the deceased are facilitated by society's expectation and permission to grieve. The individual recalls the experience of the death or loss, and remembers life as it was with the deceased. Also, during this time, the griever experiences and understands more fully the role the deceased played in his/her life. It is important for the griever to have support at this time of need.

The task of adjusting to an environment without the deceased is referred to as grief work. During this process of reconstituting a life without that person, the griever needs to re-establish social contacts, to maintain existing contacts, and to learn to function without the lost one. It is this specific task of grief work that is particularly well facilitated by self-help groups, widow/widower support groups or by such groups as the chronic obstructive lung disease group, the stroke recovery group or the amputee group. Such groups enable the individual to learn to live without the departed, whether the departed is a body function, a body part, or a loved one. Grief work is both an emotional and an instrumental task. For example, a new widow will have to learn how to cope with feelings of aloneness as well as how to change a light bulb and a new amputee will have to learn how to walk on a Terry Fox artificial leg and also how to cope with not being a physically whole person.

The final task of re-investing in a new relationship as meaningful as the lost one seems to many grievers both an enormous difficulty and evidence of disloyalty to the departed. An individual who has lost a vital body function/part may experience re-investment in the new function/part as a betrayal of one's real self. However, unless this task is accomplished, the individual will not be able to move on from the loss to regain patterns of normal, meaningful living. This particular task involves both resocialization with new partners and new patterns of living and moving toward an identity as a new person. This final task is facilitated by permitting new relationships to develop and by encouraging and supporting the necessary processes. Individuals should be encouraged to develop new skills and to experiment with different socialization. The group process offers support and socialization practice concurrently.

Research on grief over the past 25 years has demonstrated that the duration of grief depends on a number of variables. The most important variable is the success of the grief work. Clinical experience indicates that when the mourner can respond to condolences gratefully without a flood of tears, the tasks of grief are being accomplished.

THOSE AT RISK

A number of factors have been identified that place individuals at risk for abnormal grief. Any individual at risk becomes a priority for facilitation of his/her grief. (See also Chapter 4.)

The following variables define those who may be at greatest risk of experiencing an abnormal grieving process:

1. The very old and the very young
2. Same age now as significant other who died in the past
3. Physical illness
4. Psychiatric illness (especially earlier clinical depression)
5. Unresolved grief from an earlier loss
6. Concurrent life crisis and/or significant stressors
7. Poor or absent support systems
8. Highly ambivalent relationship with the deceased
9. Highly dependent relationship with deceased
10. An uncertain or not visualized loss (i.e. not seeing the body, lost at sea, in fire, in wars, etc.)
11. Multiple losses
12. Loss is socially unacceptable (homo or heterosexual liaison that was secret, loss by murder or suicide)
13. Loss that is socially negated (purposeful abortion)

The elderly are potentially at risk for abnormal grief reactions because of their age, their physical vulnerability, the number of losses they experience, and their diminished social supports. Caregivers need to be especially aware of the elderly at risk and consider them a priority for grief counselling.

THE GRIEF PROCESS IN THE ELDERLY

A number of differences between the grief process of younger persons and that of the elderly have been identified. There is an increasing awareness of the uniqueness of the elderly in their physical and emotional responses to all life events. The psychological and physiological reasons for the differences have not yet been fully explained. The following factors have been observed to be different between the young and the old:

1. Accomplishment of the tasks of grief generally take longer. This observation suggests that many elderly persons may not have fully resolved one loss before another is experienced. It may also be related to diminished energy to accomplish the tasks.

2. Emotional responses appear less than in younger persons, but there are more physical symptoms. This tendency to somatize emotional responses is particularly complex for the elderly with concurrent chronic illness. Another factor may be the societal expectation that the elderly, because they have experienced so many losses, must be "good at" resolution. (See also the discussion of hypochondriasis in Chapter 4.)

3. There is a tendency for more idealization of the deceased or the body function/part. It has been suggested that this may be both a result of the years of association and of the more severe impact of the loss to body and social integrity.

4. Significant other losses lead to greater social isolation than in younger persons. The physical incapacity of many elderly further inhibits reconstitution of social relationships. In addition, for many elderly women, there are simply not enough men of similar age to permit establishing new relationships.

5. There is a greater degree of hostility to living persons. Hostility to living persons is experienced by most grieving people. In the elderly, this appears to be greater and is often specific rather than general (i.e. a specific family member or professional contact). This observation is not well explored.

6. There is some evidence that the elderly person "withdraws" or "gives up" and does not proceed with the adaptation process. It could be speculated that vulnerability is so great that the task is too overwhelming. Somatization may also occur and energy is focussed on adapting to that symptom.

ABNORMAL GRIEF

Abnormal or pathological grief can be divided into delayed or absent grief and a distorted grief response. Delayed or absent grief may be related to the degree of stress that the individual can tolerate at one time. The depth of the relationship with the deceased is also a factor. A delayed grief reaction may be a conscious decision by an individual facing a number of concurrent life crises (i.e. during the World War II Holocaust). In this instance, the delay may be a psychological and physical necessity to protect the mourners. However, individuals who present with delayed or absent grief responses without evident or explained situational variables are particularly in need of professional intervention.

Those individuals who have distorted grief response are often those who have had an earlier unresolved grief reaction which is precipitated by this new loss. Often the response may be precipitated by the griever being the same age as the person who died earlier. Distorted grief responses may present as overactivity with no apparent loss, highly specific symptoms involving identification with the earlier deceased, or physical illness other than the identification symptom. Individuals may demonstrate behavioral alternatives toward relatives and friends over long time periods with resultant lasting losses of social contacts. Individuals may also display significant hostility to specific people and if they have had litigious interests during their life, this may involve legal action. The behavior of these individuals may be severely detrimental to their social and economic existence. The following are examples: sudden changes in residence, marital disharmony, inappropriate sexual behavior and financial irresponsibility. Occasionally, there may be such controlled hostility that the individuals appear "frozen". People may also demonstrate a depression during which they may be agitated and even suicidal. The risk of depression is greatest in those with a past history of depression, a relative with an affective disorder or previous suicide attempts. (See also Chapter 4 and Chapter 9.)

FACILITATING NORMAL GRIEVING

The facilitation of normal grieving can be accomplished in six to eight treatment sessions. It involves a number of highly specific attitudes and tasks for the practitioner who must understand normal and abnormal grief. It is also important that the grief counsellor has completed his/her own grief work. Individuals who are actively involved in their own grief work cannot be expected to have the emotional energy or patience to work with the elderly who are grieving. Awareness of one's own attitudes is an essential criterion for adequate facilitation of grief work. The practitioner needs to be comfortable with crying, anger, silence, and expressions of guilt. The practitioner needs to be especially aware of the presentation of somatic symptoms and other factors specific to the elderly person who is grieving.

The following is a review of the necessary therapeutic approaches. It is important that the grief counsellor both expect and permit individuals who are grieving to cry. Further, there must be a capacity to tolerate crying while remaining empathic and supportive. Many practitioners avoid the crying by well meaning but empty reassurances such as, "It will be alright". This glib response which primarily protects the practitioner from the pain of the griever is not a facilitating manoeuvre. Very often, the most important approach during the person's crying is a comforting silence—a silence with a conscious focus on how the grieving one is experiencing the grief as well as on the practitioner's own response to and interpretation of the crying.

In addition, the grief counsellor needs to learn to absorb the anger that is part of normal grief—the anger against the living, against the person who is dead, against the helplessness of the survivor and indeed, toward the practitioner. This anger can often be displaced in a highly personalized way toward those remaining in the environment and it is important that the practitioner facilitating normal grieving be able to absorb and accept that anger as nonpersonal and part of the normal grief response. The practitioner who recoils, makes excuses, down plays, or responds with hostility is not facilitative. To learn to absorb anger in a therapeutic manner is a complicated and lengthy process. Individuals who work with a number of grieving elderly people need to place a high priority on learning this task.

Guilt is a normal and common response to grief. Grievers experience a sense of responsibility for what has happened and wish to decrease their own helplessness by blaming themselves. Practitioners need to be aware that guilt may often be a result of some real or perceived misdeed or omission, but it is often only a way of the griever attempting to make some sense out of the loss or to find an explanation for what has occurred. Placating reassurance such as, "There, there dear, you did the best you could" is not appropriate. The grief counsellor must work through with the grieving persons what they did do, what they think they should have done, and what they would have done or usually did in similar situations in the past. The purpose is that they come to terms with the fact that they did what they could at the time. Placating reassurance tends to encourage grievers to withdraw and be left with the isolation of a secret sense of responsibility which they dare not tell others.

The specific tasks of facilitating normal grief are relatively simple and straight forward. The first task is to help the griever accept the reality of the loss. To do this, it is often most effective to have the griever review the events of the death or loss. "What happened?", "Where were you?", "What happened then?" ... "Then what did you do?", "Then what did you say?", "What did s/he say?" ... "Then what happened?", "What did s/he look like?".... On repeated review of the death or notification of loss, the reality becomes clearer as more details come into awareness. At the same time the griever experiences memories relating to the dead person. The reliving of the experience facilitates the integration of the reality of the loss and begins the second task.

The second task is the emancipation from the emotional ties with the deceased. Memories of the death can lead quite naturally into questions and comments about the memories of the deceased when alive and a discussion of their relationship. For example, the griever can talk about how s/he met the spouse and some events of their shared life together. In that process, many emotions are experienced and the mourner begins to see the deceased as s/he really was. Initially it may be perceived as only "saints who die". If the bereaved does not move from this idealized relationship, s/he may be unable to mourn the real person. Therefore, a discussion of the history of the relationship facilitates making the dead person real. During this time, the grief counsellor absorbs and encourages emotional reactions by such phrases as, "If it were me, I would feel", "Very often people feel...".

It is important to be able to inform the griever about commonly experienced phenomena. The griever's reports of feeling the presence or the auditory or visual appearance of the deceased can be a frightening experience if the griever does not know it is a quite common occurrence. Grieving people often talk about how difficult it is to experience the enormous variety of physical and emotional experiences and at the same time to be aware of the loss. As one woman said, "Not only have I lost my husband, but now I'm going crazy."

She had labelled as "going crazy" the normal physical and emotional experiences of grieving. Education about normal grief prevents this kind of interpretation. It is also appropriate and important for the grief counsellor to express sympathy with the mourner's sorrow.

The third task is for the mourner to adapt to an environment without the deceased. As mentioned earlier, this is facilitated by the modelling provided by others with similar experiences. Practitioners can help link the mourner with appropriate self-help groups or with individuals who are later in the adaptive process. The entire process of adapting to one's own loss is often facilitated by helping others with their losses. The grief counsellor must be careful to facilitate and teach, not take over the adjustment process. For example, teaching how to select a household plumber is facilitative, sending over your own plumber is not. The mourner needs to learn how to live without the deceased, not to be so taken care of that they do not learn.

Maintaining or restabilizing social contacts occurs both as part of learning to live without the deceased and part of making a new life. In making social contacts, the elderly often immediately transfer the relationship with a deceased spouse to their children or the most available professional person. Many practitioners learning to facilitate normal grief fall into the trap of taking onto themselves the emotional ties the bereaved had with a significant other. This is both inappropriate and ineffective—inappropriate for the practitioner and ineffective for the grieving elderly person who needs to make contacts that are appropriate and fully reciprocal. Grief counsellors may wish to do some specific skill teaching for the particular environment to which the mourner must adjust (i.e. how to do bank statements, how to change a fuse, how to find what agency is needed).

The fourth task of reinvesting in new relationships as meaningful as the lost one is often complex for the elderly. The grief counsellor needs to help the elderly mourner to make social contacts, other than family. To facilitate this, the environment, physical strength, disability and past social interests and skills must be evaluated with the mourner. The temptation for the elderly often is to use their children as a substitute for the dead spouse. Families of the elderly need to be helped to accomplish appropriate levels of attachment.

Families of the bereaved elderly often need assistance in understanding the mourner's appropriate task of making new meaningful relationships. Very often the families of the elderly are anxious and jealous of their parent moving on to new relationships. The elderly mourner often needs to learn new skills and behaviors appropriate to seeking new relationships. Support groups and interest groups may be useful to practise skills taught by the grief counsellor. The griever will need to discuss feelings of disloyalty to the deceased when finding someone who appears to be a replacement. A relationship as meaningful rather than a substitute or replacement is often a useful concept. Throughout the process of facilitating normal grieving it is important that the counsellor educate the griever about normal grieving, explain feelings, and offer the griever the opportunity to practise new behaviors and to understand the responses of society to his/her loss and to his/her grief process.

COPING & ADAPTATION TO CHRONIC ILLNESS

It has been estimated that 60 percent of people over 65 have one or more chronic illness. As age increases so do both the number and the severity of chronic illness. Old age is a "season of loss" of body function. All loss of functional activities results in emotional responses which either inhibit or enhance adaptation. Caregivers need to understand the process of all illness and of chronic illness in particular so that they can facilitate appropriate adaptation.

It is often helpful to incorporate concepts from a variety of sources to enable a comprehensive understanding of the illness experience. If all illness is viewed as a developmental process then the emotional responses can be better understood and appropriate intervention can occur. Several stages are suggested.

Pre-illness Stage

A genetic component which includes family history of physical and psychiatric illness and individual-specific arousal patterns is an important part of the precursors of disease.

Individual personality development including all early life experiences must be considered when examining the phases of illness. For many years there have been postulations about specific behavioral patterns as associates of specific diseases. Research data is non-conclusive as to cause-effect, but many theorists suggest that certain illnesses have identifiable behavioral correlates. Whether illness specific or not, the individual's personality assumes a major role in their experience of and adaptation to illness.

The immediate pre-illness responses to life events can be considered immediate correlates for later illness behavior.

Illness Onset Stage

The individual's experience of the symptom and the response to that symptom is a product of one's personality and culture. These two variables produce a mode of thinking in interpreting the symptom as illness and prescribing behavioral responses. For some elderly people the assigning of a disease label to symptoms, especially to chronic illness exacerbation symptoms, is avoided until physical status prevents this denial. Compliance/non-compliance with treatment regimes is part of assignation of meaning.

Hospital Stage

This stage is divided into the acute and convalescent phases. In the present health care system this stage may occur in more than one institution as well as in the patient's own home. The acute phase is often characterized by an intensive care unit experience. With or without that specific environment, the individual experiences severe anxiety not only about the symptoms, but also about the medical treatment and the environmental characteristics. Research into the experiences of individuals within intensive care units has demonstrated that the environment itself stimulates emotional responses that complicate the disease processes. The patient often experiences delirium as a result of the disease process, medication and other treatment and his/her own interpretation of the situation. The more vulnerable elderly experience all these states to a greater degree than younger persons. In addition, the chronically ill elderly have repeated history of such experiences which further colors their present experience.

The acute phase is characterized by sadness as well as anxiety and frequent delirium. This sadness appears to be a beginning recognition that things are not as they once were and it is also a beginning of a grief response to perceived losses.

The convalescent phase is characterized by grief as the individuals begin to integrate what has occurred and to discover what their status now is. Both physically and psychologically the persons may show conservation withdrawal as they reconstitute their physical state and while grieving, return to their earlier awareness. This convalescent phase of illness often occurs at home or in a rehabilitative or long-term care setting. But grief is the primary emotional state.

Altered Organism Stage

This is the phase of rehabilitation. If the acute phase is characterized by anxiety and delirium, the convalescent by grief, then the rehabilitation phase is characterized by worry. The process of adaptation and coping with an altered self is begun in earnest.

Moos (1976) has identified a variety of tasks of coping and adaptation that must be accomplished. They are as follows:

1. Maintain sense of personal worth.
2. Keep distress (physical and emotional) within manageable limits.
3. Maintain and/or restore relationships with significant others.
4. Enhance prospect for recovering bodily functions or enhance alternatives (i.e. learn to walk with an artificial leg).
5. Determine and then work toward an acceptable though altered life style.
6. Develop new skills and emphasize an opportunity for personal growth.
7. Communicate and demonstrate all these capacities to others.

These tasks can be facilitated by staff who are especially aware of

1. the usual response to a given illness, its stages, and time dimension and the extended time required by elderly with a chronic illness;
2. the major tasks of adaptation and typical coping strategies;
3. the need for emotional support;
4. the need for efforts to maintain and build a sense of personal competence;
5. the background and milieu factors that facilitate or hinder coping strategies; and
6. one's own responses to various illnesses and crises (stages and tasks etc.).

If elderly persons can demonstrate skills which reflect coping strategies, it is helpful. For example:

a) To find a general purpose or pattern of meaning in what has happened to them, hopefully a purpose that enhances rather than inhibits functioning.

b) To be able to deny or minimize the seriousness of the disease and its disabling sequela. By initial isolation or dissociation, often the elderly can gradually come to terms with their state.

c) To be able to seek relevant information especially from physicians. The respect the elderly have for their physician may create such a distance that they need assistance to increase their knowledge of the disease, its course, and treatment.

d) To request reassurance and emotional support from both individuals and groups. Elderly people may view such requests as unnecessary or humiliating. Learning to ask for what is necessary is an important skill acquisition.

e) To learn specific illness related procedures (i.e. sputum examination for infection in COPD, how to walk with a paralyzed leg).

f) To set concrete limited goals.

g) To rehearse alternative outcomes ("If I get worse, this is what will happen ...", "If I learn to use a walker, it will mean ...").

All of these coping strategies can be enhanced by skilled empathic helpers who have professional helpers of their own to communicate with (i.e. psychiatric consultation to nursing home staff). Self-help groups for individuals with similar disorders are as useful for diseases as for grief. For example, Stroke Recovery, Mended Hearts, Coping with Cancer, and Easy Breathers all provide models for identification. Elderly people need family counselling or individual counselling to facilitate coping. Spouses of the elderly may have special needs. Individuals with chronic disease need to resume former routines, functions, and relationships as early as possible. Maintenance of these not only facilitates emotional coping, but hastens physical rehabilitation.

Many elderly people with chronic illness need attention given to "cosmetic" deficits and changes. Facial surgery to correct drooping mouth, clothing and make-up to conceal gross disability are but a few examples. Medication to reduce symptoms is required as well as analgesics to control pain as much as possible. Too often elderly people are denied such assistance because they are not assertive enough to ask and caregivers do not ask.

The elderly with chronic illness need to be able to review their past life and to communicate their past achievements. For the severely disabled this can be accomplished by pictures, newspaper clippings, and other memorabilia around their institutional bed. For less disabled, the opportunity for oral history recordings or telling to associates who wish to hear about the "old days" and to learn the "old ways" is a chance for them to review the past. This retelling of a life history often inspires faith in the future. Keeping alive a determination to maintain a sense of "self" is fundamental to coping with chronic illness. Finally, every effort should be made to maintain hope—for the elderly sufferer and for his/her disease.

CONCLUSION

Loss is a "given" for the elderly. How well they cope and how much meaning they can derive from life depends on how well they have been able to cope and adapt to their multiple losses. There are some specific techniques available to caregivers to facilitate coping. That which is lost must be mourned. Facilitating that normal grief process is crucial to prevent complicated grief and facilitate adaptive responses. The caregiver can learn the techniques necessary.

REFERENCES AND SUGGESTED READINGS

Chase, Patterson and Kimball. 1977. "Psychosomatic Theories and Their Contributions to Chronic Illness." *Psychiatric Medicine.* New York: Brunner/Mazel Inc.

Fisher S. H. March 1961. "Psychiatric Considerations of Cerebral Vascular Disease." *The American Journal of Cardiology.* p. 379.

Garfield Charles A. (ed.) 1979. *Stress and Survival: The Emotional Realities of Life Threatening Illness.* C. V. Mosby.

Gerber I., A. Wiener, D. Battin and A. Arkin. 1975. "Brief Therapy to the Aged Bereaved." *Bereavement: Its Psychological Aspects.* Ed. Schoenberg, Gerber, Wiener, Kutscher and Peretz. New York: Columbia University Press.

Gramlich E. P. 1968. "Recognition and Management of Grief in Elderly Patients." *Geriatrics.* 23(7): 87–92.

Horowitz M. J. et al. 1980. "Pathological Grief and the Activation of Latent Self-images." *American Journal of Psychiatry.* 137: 1157–1162.

Lindemann Eric. 1944. "Symptomatology and Management of Acute Grief." *American Journal of Psychiatry.* 101: 141–149.

Moos R. H. (ed.) 1977. *Coping with Physical Illness.* Plenum Medical Book Co.

Moos R. H. (ed.) 1976. *Human Adaptation: Coping With Life Crises.* Lexington: D. Health.

Moos R. H. and V. D. Tsu. 1977. "The Crisis of Physical Illness: An Overview." *Coping With Physical Illness.* New York: Plenum Publishing Co.

Rowett D. B. and D. L. Dudley. 1978. "COPD: Psychosocial and Psychophysiological Issues." *Psychosomatics.* 19(5).

Shapiro L. N. and A. W. McMahon. 1966. "Rehabilitation Stalemate." *Archives of General Psychiatry.* 15: 173–177.

Worden J. William. 1982. *Grief Counseling and Grief Therapy.* New York: Springer Publishing Company.

3

Psychodynamics and Ageing

Donald A. Wasylenki, M.D., M.Sc., F.R.C.P.(C)

Sigmund Freud, at age 49, wrote as follows:

> The age of patients has this much importance in determining
> their fitness for psycho-analytic treatment, that, on the one hand,
> near or above the age of fifty the elasticity of the mental processes,
> on which the treatment depends, is as a rule lacking—old people
> are no longer educable—and, on the other hand, the mass of
> material to be dealt with would prolong the duration of the
> treatment indefinitely (Freud 1953).

Karl Abraham (1942), however, reported good results with elderly patients.
Fenichel's (1945) opinion was that psychoanalytic approaches with the elderly
were indicated if libidinal and narcissistic gratification could still be achieved.
Other workers have also been optimistic about possibilities for conflict resolution
in old age. Freud himself displayed very little loss of elasticity in middle and
late life. He was 44 when *The Interpretation of Dreams* was published and
81 when *Analysis Terminable and Interminable* appeared. In discussing the
last phase of Freud's life, Jones described "the truly astonishing fresh outburst
of original ideas he produced in these years, just when it was thought he had
rounded off his life's work" (1957, 243).

For many, however, and particularly for those who become our patients,
old age is a season of loss. Old age is analogous to a chronic illness. It is
a condition in which previous functional efficiency has been lost and the capacity
for restitution progressively impaired. Any change in life that requires in-depth
re-adjustment may cause psychological dysfunction if the re-adjustment fails.
In old age the individual is confronted with new and specific problems such
as declining physical abilities, illness, lost reproductive function, retirement,
loneliness due to the death of a spouse, relatives and friends, and the awareness
of approaching death itself. Much psychopathology can be understood as a
reaction to these cumulative losses. Difficulties are most severe in people who

have not succeeded in resolving earlier conflicts. Unfortunately, there is a strong tendency to attribute emotional disorder in the elderly to organic factors, affective disorders, or vague concepts such as senility. Too often this leads to therapeutic nihilism or exclusive reliance on physical methods of treatment. This chapter presents three cases that illustrate common psychodynamic themes and emphasize the importance of psychological understanding.

MR. M.—REDISTRIBUTION OF LIBIDO

Mr. M. was a 78 year old retired manufacturer, married, with two daughters and three grandchildren. He had postponed retirement until age 76, when he and his partner sold their business. He came for treatment because of a strong desire to leave his wife after 48 years of marriage. He sought advice from an acquaintance who was a social worker and she referred him for psychotherapy. He had been seen by a psychiatrist one year earlier, diagnosed as depressed, and treated unsuccessfully with antidepressants. Since retiring he had lost his enthusiasm for life. He had always dealt with emptiness and loneliness by losing himself in his work. Now he felt useless and discarded. Much of his dissatisfaction focussed on his wife. He complained that she was uninterested in him and that she provided no love or affection. He had realized early on that their marriage was a mistake. He had wanted to marry her sister because "she was more lively and more witty—better company." He had "settled" for his wife and soon became too absorbed in developing his manufacturing business to spend time with his family. Now he resented that his wife continued to pursue her own interests and was unavailable to him. ("She won't even hold me when I ask her to.") He believed that his wife, daughters and sons-in-law were contemptuous of his weakened state. At times, looking in the mirror at night, he felt extreme panic and would shout out some expletive. Then, unable to sleep, he would ruminate over his past failures.

He was the youngest in a sibship of six and grew up in a poor neighborhood in Montreal. His father was "a scholar" who spent most of his time in a synagogue. He was contemptuous of his father for having been a weak man and a poor provider. He idealized his mother, describing her as a strong woman who was very good to everyone. She had nursed him through osteomyelitis and as the youngest child he had always felt a special relationship to her.

He was portly and well groomed, dressed in a suit and tie as if going to work. He tried to conceal a slight hearing loss. He was irritable and expressed considerable hostility towards his wife. He believed that if only he could escape from her, all would be restored to him. Although he complained of diminished memory and powers of concentration, formal testing revealed no deficits. His mood was depressed and he admitted to fleeting thoughts of suicide.

There is much to be learned about the impact of retirement on the individual. Epidemiological studies have failed to demonstrate negative effects. However, it is generally agreed that for some, perhaps 10 percent, retirement does cause considerable distress. Those most at risk appear to be people whose work has been highly cathected with narcissistic libido, that is, those for whom work has been the most important, often the exclusive source of feelings of competence, strength, self-regard, and self-esteem. Even in those who have achieved a better libidinal balance the self-depleting impact of retirement may be manifested in milder form. In a sample of 20 schoolteachers interviewed one year after retirement, 9 reported stereotypical work-related dreams in which the retiree was a teacher again. The dreamer was filled with anxiety because he was no longer able to teach. Either he had arrived late, or the students ignored him, or he was unprepared or unable to locate his classroom. Talking about these dreams invariably revealed feelings of weakness and lost competence.

Mr. M. clearly had made an excessive libidinal investment in his work. Loss of work was a significant narcissistic loss for which he was initially unable to make restitution. He described a compelling image of himself after retiring. While he had worked, even at an advanced age, he had felt strong, agile, and attractive, "like a shiny fly in the summertime, impossible to catch." After retirement he felt weak, slow, and dull, "like a fly in winter, waiting to be squashed." He attempted to make restitution by turning to his wife, after 48 years of ignoring her, and became enraged when his demands were frustrated, adding further to the narcissistic trauma. Meissner (1978) has described how such trauma may lead to feelings of depression and depletion resulting in the development of defensive paranoid trends. Mr. M.'s criticism and blaming of his wife and family and his eventual desire for disengagement from them appeared to be manifestations of this mechanism.

Mr. M. described his life as boring and himself as apathetic. He spent most of his time reading and "going downtown." Levin (1965) suggests that this state often arises in the elderly due to difficulty in mobilizing drive behavior. In fact, he understands much of the psychological difficulty in old age as a problem of redistribution of libido. With retirement, Mr. M. was faced with the necessity of redistributing a large quantity of both narcissistic and object libido. The suddenness of the demand and the large quantity of libido involved led to maladaptive responses. He became excessively self-absorbed. Attempts to re-engage his wife were based on an unrealistic assessment of her availability maintained through the use of denial. His persistent focussing on his marriage as the only possible source of substitute gratification blocked his ability to consider other avenues for redistribution. This focussing was abetted by castration anxiety (fear that in his weakened state he would no longer be able to perform genitally) and the need to reassert sexual potency with his wife. He expressed concern over the diminished amount of semen he produced when he masturbated.

Mr. M. was seen in semiweekly psychotherapy for eight months. The goal was to help him achieve a more satisfactory and age-appropriate redistribution of both object and narcissistic libido. This, it was felt, would reduce his frustration and rage, ameliorate his feelings of depression and emptiness, and attenuate his drive to act out by ending his marriage.

Levin (1978) suggests that the maintenance of narcissistic libido in the elderly can be thought of in terms of the past, the present, and the future.

Mr. M.'s attachment to his past experience was intense but it was not in the service of enhancing self esteem. Rather it was an unrealistic and grandiose elaboration of past victories and ventures. Because his narcissistic aspirations remained the same at age 76 as they had been at 30 or 40, this maladaptive reminiscence served only to remind him of the gap between ego ideal and present reality. This would alternate with ruminations about past failures, emphasizing the defensive nature of his grandiosity. Thus, at the beginning of therapy, past experience was unavailable to him as a source of self-esteem and satisfaction.

Mr. M.'s attitudes toward the present were also maladaptive. Because of his high aspirations, he was unable to consider any new form of activity. As an extremely successful businessperson, he was recognized as a source of valuable advice and information. However, he regarded any position that entailed a decrease in direct performance or control as unsatisfactory. He was unable to shift from one level of aspiration to another—from generativity to ego integrity, in Erikson's (1975) terms. Present satisfaction should also have been attainable through relationships with his children and grandchildren. Although he had invested little in his family in earlier life he now felt drawn towards them. Again, however, he was blocked by the projection of his own feelings of weakness and self-contempt into his daughters and their husbands. He was convinced that "the younger generation" harbored hostility towards him.

In terms of the future, religious belief can be an important means of maintaining narcissistic equilibrium in old age. Mr. M. had always been interested in religion. He emphasized that he was not one of those "idiots" who actually believed in God and in an afterlife but he did have an academic interest in religion. He liked to read about it and to debate with "true believers," as he called several of his friends. The restriction of his religious self seemed to be related to strong negative feelings about his father's investment in religion.

Much of the psychotherapy with Mr. M. was a reactivation of the past. Butler calls this approach "life review therapy" (1963). It is an attempt to enhance a universal mental process in the elderly characterized by the progressive return to consciousness of past experiences, particularly those involving unresolved conflicts. Mr. M.'s reminiscence had taken on a pathological quality. As his view of the past became more realistic, several things began to happen. First, there was discomfort as he became aware of the grandiosity of his view. This was followed by more realistic satisfaction with his considerable successes and acceptance of his various failures. This enabled him to disengage from the past and begin to develop a less stringent ego-ideal that allowed him to seek substitute satisfactions in the present.

He accepted several consulting jobs, advising people who were starting small businesses, and he was surprised to find that he felt satisfied and fulfilled despite not being in full control. Berezin (1978) has described achievement of the "consultative position" as the essential developmental task in old age. He notes, "The consultative position implies that the aged person, by reason of having lived and survived a full life, has profited in experience, training, discrimination, judgment, wisdom and the like. By virtue of such achievements, he is now available to help others, as an objective philosopher, as it were" (Berezin 1978, 106). Berezin sees the consultative phase as a continuation of the generative stage without the accompanying responsibility. He suggests that it may, in a special way, be a replacement for lost genital primacy. As Mr.

M. attained this position it became obvious in the transference. He began to enquire about the therapist's financial affairs and to offer suggestions on financial management.

The transference relationship reactivated object libido. Disengagement became re-engagement first in the transference and then in the outside world. This was facilitated by the therapist's willingness to acknowledge and discuss sexual fantasies, experiences, and wishes. Initially Mr. M. had felt that a young man would be contemptuous of the persistence of sexuality in an old man in addition to the loss of productivity through work. With a gain in narcissistic supplies through consulting work and a gain in libidinal attachment in the transference, Mr. M.'s self-esteem improved considerably. This allowed him to establish more satisfactory relationships with his family. He was also able to work through aspects of his relationship with his father and use his interest in religion to further elaborate his self-image. At the end of therapy he reported feeling more equanimity. The desire to end his marriage had receded, his increased alcohol consumption had diminished, and he had even obtained a hearing aid.

MRS. S.—OBJECTIVE ANXIETY

Mrs. S. was 70 years old, Jewish, and married with no children. She had worked as a milliner until she was 60, when both she and her husband retired. They lived in an older section of the city that had changed from Jewish to Italian/Portuguese. Mrs. S. had no previous psychiatric contacts. She presented with a six-month history of anxiety, anorexia, insomnia, confusion, and dizziness. Extensive medical and neurological investigation, including EEG and CAT scan, were all negative. The most striking feature of her presentation was severe anxiety. Her main concern was "What is going to happen to me?" She was afraid to go out by herself. She was especially frightened at night and she complained that no one could help her. Her husband, who suffers from Buerger's disease, had been gradually immobilized by pain in his legs. Mrs. S.'s difficulties developed when her husband was scheduled for surgery. She was afraid that he would not be available to comfort her if she awoke feeling upset, and that they would be sent to live out their lives alone in separate institutions.

Her history revealed a lifelong pattern of dependency. She was born in Russia. Her mother was an invalid and Mrs. S. remembered people coming in to do the housework. She was "spoiled" by her three older brothers and her father and never did any work in the home. She married a man who was devoted to her. She had always felt close to her husband and dependent on him. He described her as nervous, dependent, and passive, but warm and competent until the onset of her symptoms.

When first seen she was extremely agitated. She paced about, wringing her hands. She complained of dizziness, spots in front of her eyes, and feelings of dread. At times she would shout out her husband's name or pound on the wall. She felt ashamed of this and was afraid she was losing her mind. She constantly sought reassurance that "someone will look after me." She denied feelings of guilt or sadness and suicidal ideation. There was no evidence of cognitive impairment. Initially she was hospitalized, diagnosed as suffering from a late life depression and treated with tricyclic antidepressants and major tranquillizers. There was no improvement. Eventually she was managed as an outpatient with brief, regular psychotherapy, minimal home support, and diazepam 5 mg HS.

The key to Mrs. S.'s management lay in the nature of her extreme anxiety. Freud defined anxiety as the central problem of neuroses. The prototype, traumatic anxiety, occurs at birth and at other times in early infancy when the immature ego is overwhelmed by stimuli. This forms the basis of the ego's perception of danger throughout adult life. Signal anxiety is an attenuated form of anxiety that occurs when danger is anticipated. This instinctual anxiety is characteristic of adult neuroses and has been defined as dread of the strength of the instincts. It enables the ego to activate defense mechanisms to inhibit impulses. Anna Freud (1966) points out that the ego in the developing child defends not only against dangerous instincts but also against outside threats. The greater the importance of the outside world as a source of security and protection, the more likely anxiety is to arise from that source. This has been called objective anxiety. When one is too weak to actively oppose the outside world—to defend against it or modify it—then objective anxiety may become severe.

Zetzel (1962) suggests that the elderly, like the very young, typically experience anxiety not in relation to internal danger but in relation to something external. Elderly people who are dependent on others are prone to this type of anxiety, which is often stimulated by fear of loss or separation. Goldfarb (1953) states that what is feared is loss of the material implications of personal relationships. The fear is not so much loss of love as loss of those who can provide and protect. Anxiety in response to threatened loss is more often a result of actual circumstances than a signal of instinctual danger. It usually has a depressive quality. The prevalence of this more primitive form of anxiety in old age is consistent with a developmental psychology which includes both progressive and regressive directions. As the cumulative strain of ageing lessened Mrs. S.'s capacity to cope with her husband's anticipated disability, anxieties from an earlier developmental level became more prominent. Early object relations, in particular a maladaptive identification with her invalid mother, contributed to the intensity of this episode. Once this was understood, strategies for management became clear.

Mrs. S. also showed structural modifications characteristic of many elderly patients. Although the id, ego, and superego maintain their distinctive attributes throughout life, in old age a new homeostasis may develop. Shifts in homeostasis have been commented on by Zinberg and Kaufman (1978) and others. Since the impulses contained in the id are timeless the process of ageing does not change them. What may occur is a more direct expression of libidinal and aggressive drives. The aim of the impulses may be somewhat altered but there are fewer inhibitions on expression. Mrs. S. did not attempt to cajole her family or friends into helping her or use some other rational means of obtaining increased support. Rather she shouted her husband's name, reiterated her needs ("Who's going to help me?"), and expressed her frustration by pounding on the walls. Although she was frightened by these discharge phenomena, she reported feelings of calm and decreased anxiety afterwards, "like relaxing after a storm." A developmental concept in psychoanalysis is that primitive impulses are partially tamed by gradual fusion of libidinal and aggressive components. In ageing there may be a gradual defusion which permits greater direct expression. In order to maintain self-esteem in the face of anticipated and experienced losses in old age, the ego becomes more concerned with obtaining narcissistic supplies. This is often facilitated by some lifting of repression.

Regression may serve the same function in the elderly that repression does in youth. Regression as a defense may allow the elderly person to find dependency relationships that are adaptive and conflict-free. In Mrs. S.'s case, however, the regression was maladaptaive. She felt helpless and overwhelmed by anxiety and her demands to be taken care of could not be satisfied by her interpersonal environment.

Denial related to threats from the outside world is a common defense mechanism in the elderly. Mrs. S. utilized a particular form of denial—ego restriction—to avoid experiences and perceptions that reminded her of her losses and helplessness. This resulted in the loss of important functions. She became unable to cook and prepare meals ("That's funny, I just seem to forget") lest she have difficulties that would remind her of her dependency ("Joe always used to help me."). After her husband's below-knee amputation she was unable to help with the bandaging and stump care because looking at the amputated limb reminded her of her husband's loss of strength as a protective figure. She tried to ward off disagreeable external stimuli, but at the price of increased helplessness.

The need for direct narcissistic supplies in old age seems to override earlier, more strict superego demands. The need to obtain love, affection, protection, and security from figures in the environment makes their reactions, and perhaps those of earlier parental figures, more important than later identifications organized as conscience. This degree of superego weakening contributed to lifting of repression and direct instinctual expression in Mrs. S. She was able to make direct demands of her environment without feeling guilt or shame.

The approach to therapy with Mrs. S. was based on recognition of the objective quality of her anxiety. She was desperately searching for some security in the face of feelings of helplessness and fear as she anticipated the loss of the one person who protected and provided for her. Inability to master intense anxiety, which was exacerbated by earlier conflicts around dependency, undermined her self-esteem and increased her vulnerability. What was required was not interpretive intervention but a concrete and stable protective relationship. This was established initially by weekly contacts along with availability by telephone, and eventually by brief monthly contacts with some homecare involvement.

Goldfarb (1955) has described the mechanism of this approach to psychotherapy with the elderly. He believes that the panic experienced by subjectively helpless elderly people can be rapidly attenuated by a relationship with a therapist seen as a parent-surrogate, protector and provider. The fostering of the illusion of direct aid rather than assistance in helping oneself increases self-esteem. As the elderly patient becomes convinced of his/her good standing with the powerful therapist, self-regard mounts and the sense of helplessness subsides.

Once Mrs. S. sensed that her feelings of need and expectation for care would not be frustrated by the parent-therapist she was able to begin to develop mastery. In particular, there was a marked diminution in anxiety and ego restriction and she began to experiment with more adaptive solutions, e.g., attendance at a day centre. As the therapist continued to admire and support her improvements, her ability to function effectively gradually returned to a pre-morbid level. With this improvement a mild elevator phobia, which had disappeared during her crisis state, reappeared, suggesting a return to more mature neurotic mechanisms. Although this approach to therapy does not present significant curative potential, it did allow Mrs. S. to develop techniques of environmental mastery. This enhanced her self-esteem and contributed to feelings of self-mastery which will sustain her in dealing with inevitable future losses.

MR. B.—REHABILITATION FAILURE

Mr. B. was a 68 year old retired salesperson, married with one son. He had sustained a left hemiplegia following a cerebrovascular accident six months before. Following his stroke Mr. B. had been admitted to an acute care hospital where he received a short course of rehabilitation. He refused transfer to a stroke rehabilitation unit and was discharged home. Before the stroke he had been extremely active but on his return from the hospital his wife described him as "a different person." He became housebound and refused to see his friends or relatives, saying, "No one wants to see me like this." In fact, his hemiplegia was relatively mild and he had only slight facial paralysis. He became extremely demanding of his wife; all her time was devoted to him. She had to attend to every detail of his meals, his dress, his comfort and his toilet. He constantly sought reassurance that she still loved him and would stay with him. As he began to lose many of the gains he had made, his wife became more concerned.

Finally, he was persuaded to enter the hospital for more rehabilitation. The hospital staff quickly grew irritated and alienated by his constant demands and complaints. At times he was despondent and said he would rather be dead than crippled. He would lie in bed for long periods refusing to eat or speak and refusing rehabilitation. It was at this point that his attending physician diagnosed depression and requested a psychiatric consultation.

Mr. B. was the eldest of three, with two sisters. His father left the family when the patient was eleven. He completed high school and then went to work to help support the family. He did this for a number of years and contributed money to his sisters' education. He married a woman ten years younger and refused to allow her to work. He became a very successful insurance salesperson and won several sales awards. When his mother was disabled by a stroke he arranged for her nursing home care and visited her regularly until she died. Following retirement he became active as a volunteer with several organizations for the disabled.

When first seen on the stroke rehabilitation unit, he was sitting in a wheelchair and seldom moved his left arm. He was critical of hospital routines and pessimistic about prospects for recovery. There was little evidence of cognitive impairment. He explained his despondency by saying, "How would you feel if you were in my position?" He said that he often wished he were dead but never thought of committing suicide.

To help Mr. B. it was necessary to understand the psychological mechanisms underlying his response to his disability. Any major traumatic event occurring without warning will produce profound psychological regression. Usually the patient's own healing forces and the protective atmosphere of the hospital promote recovery from the initial state of disruption. This is followed by a sequence of reactions to physical illness including first temporarily increased dependency, then grief during the convalescent period, next mastery of adaptive tasks in the rehabilitative period and finally, gradual recognition and acceptance of the extent of the disability. Mr. B. had been unable to navigate this psychological course. The need to become dependent due to a real limitation had activated earlier feelings of helplessness and revived old problems around dependency. Much of Mr. B.'s life had been a reaction against basic dependent needs. He had never been able to allow himself any degree of legitimate dependency. He had developed a pseudo-independent lifestyle, masking underlying dependency wishes with apparent self-sufficiency. When the stroke disrupted his capacity to "do for himself", he used very primitive ways of dealing with his feelings of helplessness and unwanted wishes to be cared for. His inability to accept enforced dependency blocked the normal grieving process that is necessary before the tasks of rehabilitation can be undertaken.

Underlying and intensifying Mr. B.'s conflict with dependency were intense narcissistic concerns. He was attempting to determine whether his wife and family, and later the hospital staff, could possibly value him in his crippled and dependent state. It was as if he were trying to restore his shattered self-esteem by using his family's and the staff's view of him as a person worth caring for. The predominant orientation of his relationships became self-concern, self-gratification, and self-preservation—direct expressions of narcissistic needs. Any delay or disappointment in meeting these needs was experienced as further trauma, leading to rage, anxiety, and feelings of helplessness. As mentioned earlier, narcissistic rage is often projected, resulting in alienation of the very people the regressed, traumatized person is most dependent on. This pattern is too familiar in chronic care and rehabilitation hospitals and often leads to failure in rehabilitation.

Mr. B. expressed many anxieties common to stroke patients. Chief among these was the fear that he would be left crippled and dependent on others for things he had previously taken for granted. This was somewhat inconsistent with the progress he had made in the first month of rehabilitation. He considered himself an unwelcome burden to himself and his family. He was afraid that he would suffer another stroke and was convinced that this would mean the end of him. He was frightened that his money would be used up in paying for eventual institutional care.

A central task leading to acceptance of disablity is a reorganization of the composite picture the person has of his body so that the deformed part can somehow be fitted into his image of himself. The key obstacle to this reintegration is the mechanism of denial. Beneath Mr. B.'s feelings of helplessness and despondency lay a refusal to recognize the permanence of his disability. Denial and regression were his main defense mechanisms against post-stroke anxieties. He also strongly resisted psychiatric consultation. His energy seemed entirely focussed on his physical handicap and he vehemently denied any suggestion that he might be having emotional difficulties.

Psychotherapeutic work with Mr. B. was done via the staff on the rehabilitation unit. The major aims were to help him overcome his denial, to support him as he experienced the normal depression characteristic of grief in the convalescent period, and to provide him with some insight into his problems with dependency. In addition, his wife was seen by the unit social worker. She expressed anxiety about leaving her husband alone when he was home on weekends. This led to a tendency to overprotect, which exacerbated his regressive behavior. She was encouraged to allow him to maintain his previous dominant role in family decision-making as much as possible. He had shown signs of relinquishing this completely when he first returned home. As a result of this management plan, Mr. B.'s attitudes and behavior changed significantly and his rehabilitation progressed rapidly, following a period of normal depression.

It is essential that staff, who deal with elderly patients disabled by chronic or catastrophic illnesses, understand the normal stages of illness development. In the convalescent phase, which begins with some stabilization in the patient's condition, grief reactions are precipitated by acknowledgment of disability. Anger, guilt, and depression are common features and staff members should be helped to tolerate the expression of these affects without labelling the patient emotionally ill or unco-operative. Staff may become the recipients of projected anger or guilt and they often need to be primed to endure. When regressive manifestations such as denial and dependency conflicts are prolonged, staff members need to be able to confront patients in an atmosphere of support and concern. Staff members must also understand the tasks of coping and adaptation characteristic of the rehabilitative phase. During this phase the work of grief is replaced by the work of worry. Patients begin to develop more realistic concerns about whether they will be able to function in a disabled state and whether they will be accepted by others. Essential to this phase is the presence of staff members who relate to the patient as a person rather than just as a patient. During this phase in particular, it is important that staff allow patients to develop independent functioning. It is also crucial for staff to understand their own reactions to particular types of disabling and disfiguring illnesses in order to work effectively with patients such as Mr. B.

CONCLUSION

These three cases demonstrate the importance of psychological observation and psychodynamic understanding in working with the elderly. It is particularly important to recognize and understand the vicissitudes of regression. Regression may be adaptive in the service of the ego, or pathological in severe disturbances such as schizophrenia. In old age, when accustomed sources of gratification become unavailable, some regression is both necessary and adaptive. The degree of regression and the ability of the older person to accept regression, which is determined by earlier conditions, often determine the quality of the last stage of the life cycle.

When regression becomes severe or when it leads to reactivation of earlier conflicts, older patients are often misdiagnosed. Dementia and delirium are relatively easy to rule out by means of a careful mental status examination with or without psychological testing. It is much more difficult to rule out depression. Goldfarb (1978) has contributed some useful observations on this point. Although such patients often appear depressed this is not an accurate description of their mood. They are more often anxious (Mrs. S.) or angry (Mr. M.). There is a tendency to externalize: the environment is attacked or blamed, often in a frankly paranoid fashion. There is little evidence of guilt. Suicidal ideation is rare. There is a passive wish to be dead, but various reasons are given for not committing suicide. Finally there is a total lack of joy—a quality of anhedonia—which Goldfarb (1978) understands as a means of guaranteeing care from a world experienced as desolate and deserted.

These three cases illustrate common issues in dealing with elderly patients. They possessed few of the factors looked for in selecting patients for psychotherapy. Mrs. S. was far from physically attractive. She seemed intellectually impoverished, and although she was verbal she was certainly not articulate. Initially she posed a direct threat to the therapist's yearnings for omnipotence by seeming to grow worse instead of better. Her obvious desire to be helped rather than to learn to help herself was also difficult to accept. Working with these patients stimulated conflicts in the therapist related to his own parents. The therapist also felt that the patients, particularly Mr. M. and Mr. B., would be unwilling to trust someone younger than themselves. On the other hand, there was a sense of urgency in the therapy with Mr. M. that helped develop a more productive therapeutic alliance. This may have been due to feelings that this was a last chance to make some significant alteration in his life. In all three cases the lessening of repression allowed for easier access to memories and associations which provided useful insight into earlier conflicts and experiences. Treatment of these patients, undertaken with some trepidation, turned out to be highly gratifying. The universal human tendency towards conflict resolution and mastery persisted and became the basis for effective therapeutic management.

REFERENCES AND SUGGESTED READINGS

Abraham K. 1942. *The Applicability of Psychoanalytic Treatment to Patients of Advanced Age: Selected Papers.* London: Hogarth Press.

Berezin M. 1978. "Some Intrapsychic Aspects of Aging." Ed. N. E. Zinberg and I. Kaufman. *Normal Psychology of the Aging Process.* New York: International Universities Press.

Bibring C. 1966. "Old Age: Its Liabilities and Its Assets: A Psychobiological Discourse." *Psychoanalysis: A General Psychology.* Ed. R. M. Loewenstein et al. New York: International Universities Press.

Butler R. N. 1963. "The Life Review: An Interpretation of Reminiscence in the Aged." *Psychiatry.* 26: 65–76.

Cath S. H., K. E. Gluck and H. T. Blane. 1957. "The Role of the Body-Image in Psychotherapy with the Physically Handicapped." *Psychoanalytic Review.* 44: 34–40.

Erickson E. 1975. *Childhood and Society.* New York: W. W. Norton.

Fenichel O. 1945. *The Psychoanalytic Theory of Neurosis.* New York: W. W. Norton.

Freud A. 1966. *The Ego and the Mechanisms of Defense.* New York: International Universities Press.

Freud S. 1953. *On Psychotherapy, Standard Edition.* Vol. 7. London: Hogarth Press. p. 257.

Goldfarb A. 1978. "A Psychosocial and Sociophysiological Approach to Aging." *Normal Psychology of the Aging Process.* Ed. N. E. Zinberg and I. Kaufman. New York: International Universities Press.

Goldfarb A. 1955. "Psychotherapy of Aged Persons IV: One Aspect of the Psychodynamics of the Therapeutic Situation with Aged Patients." *Psychoanalytic Review.* 42: 180–187.

Goldfarb A. and H. Turner. 1953. "Psychotherapy of Aged Persons II: Utilization and Effectiveness of Brief Therapy." *American Journal of Psychiatry.* 109: 916–921.

Grotjohn M. 1955. "Analytic Psychotheraphy With the Elderly." *Psychoanalytic Review.* 42: 419.

Jones E. 1957. *The Life and Work of Sigmund Freud Vol. 3: The Last Phase: 1919–1939.* New York: Basic Books.

Kimball C. P. 1977. "Psychosomatic Theories and Their Contributions to Chronic Illness." *Psychiatric Medicine.* Ed. G. Usdin. New York: Bruner Mazel.

Levin S. 1978. "Libido Equilibrium." *Normal Psychology of the Aging Process.* Ed. N. E. Zinberg and I. Kaufman. New York: International Universities Press.

Levin S. 1965. "Some Comments on the Distribution of Narcissistic and Object Libido in the Aged." *International Journal of Psychoanalysis.* 46: 200–208.

Meissner W. W. 1978. "Discussion of Social Learning and Self-Image in Aging by N. E. Zinberg." *Normal Psychology of the Aging Process.* Ed. N. E. Zinberg and I. Kaufman. New York: International Universities Press.

Segal H. 1955. "Fear of Death: Notes on the Analysis of an Old Man." *International Journal of Psychoanalysis.* 39: 170.

Wasylenki D. 1980. *Retirement and Psychosocial Stress.* Master's Thesis. Institute of Medical Sciences. University of Toronto.

Wasylenki D. and A. MacBride. 1981. "Retirement." *Modern Perspectives in the Psychiatry of Middle Age.* Ed. J. G. Howells. New York: Bruner Mazel.

Zetzel E. R. 1962. "Dynamics of the Metapsychology of the Aging Process." *Geriatric Psychiatry.* Ed. M. A. Berezin & S. H. Cath. New York: International Universities Press.

Zinberg N. E. and I. Kaufman. 1978. "Cultural and Personality Factors Associated with Aging: An Introduction." *Normal Psychology of the Aging Process.* Ed. N. E. Zinberg and I. Kaufman. New York: International Universities Press.

Part Two
CLINICAL SYNDROMES

4

Depression

Donald A. Wasylenki, M.D., M.Sc., F.R.C.P. (C)

Depression accounts for the majority of late life mental disorders. Suicide increases with age and depression and suicide in this group are major public health problems which will escalate as the elderly population expands.

Depression may refer to a mood, a symptom or a syndrome. Depressed mood describes feelings of sadness, disappointment, discouragement and related emotions. Depression as a symptom refers to mood changes associated with other psychiatric disorders, medical diseases, or drug effects. The syndrome of depression consists of cognitive, affective, vegetative, and motor components. Affect may be despairing and hopeless. Thought processes are slow, and thought content is morbid and guilt-ridden. Appetite, sleep, weight, and energy are disturbed, and the patient shows either agitated or retarded motor behavior. The classical depressive triad consists of sadness, difficulty in thinking, and motor retardation.

Table 4.1 shows the American Psychiatric Association's criteria for a major depressive episode. At least four major symptoms must be present along with dysphoric mood. There are further subclassifications of the depressive syndrome (e.g., primary/secondary, unipolar/bipolar, pure depressive disease/depressive spectrum disease) which may be of considerable research significance, but which are not critical for this discussion.

The importance of recognizing these signs and symptoms lies in the fact that with appropriate treatment, depressive syndromes have a favorable prognosis. Approximately 80 percent of persons with a depressive syndrome will respond to antidepressant medication in one to four weeks. This percentage may be somewhat lower in elderly patients. Studies have also demonstrated the efficacy of psychotherapy alone and in combination with pharmacotherapy for acute ambulatory depressives. The major difficulty lies in recognizing and providing treatment for depressive syndromes in the elderly. Figure 4.1 shows rates of treatment by age, for persons with a major or minor depression. Treatment was very broadly defined, but even within a broad definition, there is a marked decrease in the percentage of persons receiving treatment after age 56. These trends were the same for both men and women.

TABLE 4.1

Diagnostic Criteria for Major Depressive Episode

A. Dysphoric mood or loss of interest or pleasure in all or almost all usual activities and pastimes.

B. At least four of the following symptoms:
   (1) poor appetite and significant weight loss or increased appetite and significant weight gain.
   (2) insomnia or hypersomnia.
   (3) psychomotor agitation or retardation.
   (4) loss of interest or pleasure in usual activities, or decrease in sexual drive not limited to a period when delusional or hallucinating.
   (5) loss of energy; fatigue.
   (6) feelings of worthlessness, self-reproach, or excessive or inappropriate guilt.
   (7) complaints or evidence of diminished ability to think or concentrate.
   (8) recurrent thoughts of death, suicidal ideation, wishes to be dead, or suicide attempt.

These symptoms must occur in the absence of bizarre pre-morbid behavior, schizophrenic, paranoid or organic mental disorder, or uncomplicated bereavement.

American Psychiatric Association Diagnostic and Statistical Manual of Mental Disorders, Third Edition. Washington, DC, copyright APA 1980. Used with permission.

FIGURE 4.1

Treatment for Emotional Problems during the Past Year Among Subjects with Current Major or Minor Depression

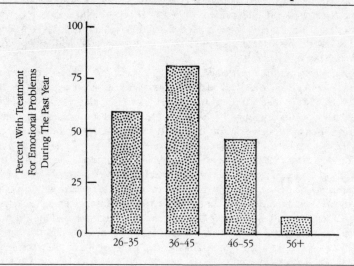

Weissman M. M. and J. K. Myers. 1979. "Depression in the Elderly: Research Directions in Psychopathology, Epidemiology and Treatment." *Journal of Geriatric Psychiatry.* 12: 187-201.

FREQUENCY AND DISTRIBUTION

Epidemiological information about depression is unreliable because of methodological difficulties such as case definition and identification. However, depressive syndromes are the most common of all major mental disorders and the average prevalence worldwide is three to four percent. In the elderly it is closer to 10 percent.

Figure 4.2 shows findings for rates of major and minor depression for both men and women. Overall rates are higher in women than in men, but women's rates are higher only up to age 55. After age 55 men catch up. While the rates appear to drop after age 75, one cannot be sure about this as data are incomplete. The patterns outlined—higher rates in younger women, a plateau with age in women and increase with age in men—have been reported in several studies.

FIGURE 4.2

Current Prevalence Rates per 100 of Major or Minor Depression

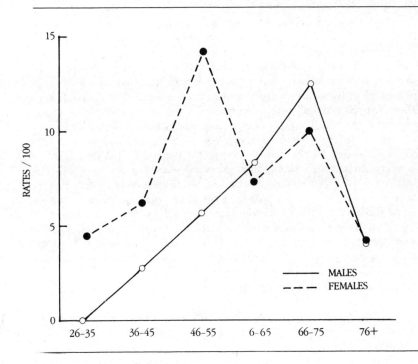

Weissman M. M and J. K. Myers. 1979. "Depression in the Elderly: Research Directions in Psychopathology, Epidemiology and Treatment." *Journal of Geriatric Psychiatry.* 12: 187–201.

There is a close relationship between significant physical illness and depression in old age. Thirty to fifty percent of elderly patients with physical disease suffer from concomitant depression.

Mild depressions, which are sometimes also early depressions, are very common in the elderly. Forty to fifty percent of elderly community residents complain of transient, recurring disturbances of mood. These episodes may last from a few minutes to a few days, and are characterized by feelings of discouragement, uselessness, and sometimes by a passive wish for a painless death.

To complete the epidemiological picture, suicide rates increase dramatically with age. The suicide rate in Canada for males over 65 is 30 to 40/100 000 compared with the general population rate of 12.6/100 000. Whereas many more young people attempt than commit suicide, among the elderly the ratio is only 2 to 3 to 1. The diagnosis of depression carries an annual suicide rate of 551/100 000 in those over 55, compared with 159/100 000 for those under 55.

CLINICAL FEATURES

Age changes occur in the form and content of depressive disorders. Depressions in the elderly are increasingly severe, more protracted, and recur with increasing frequency. As a rule, agitation is more common in older and retardation in younger depressed patients. Also, the tendency to be concerned with bodily functions and contents increases with rising age, and in 40 to 50 percent of elderly depressed patients, hypochondriasis is a prominent feature. These hypochondriacal complaints frequently obscure the presence of real physical illness which so commonly accompanies depression in this age group.

There has been some confusion regarding the relationship of organic cerebral changes and late life depression. In the past, it has been felt that brain changes might account for an increased vulnerability to depressive disorder. However, it has been established that late life depressions and dementia are quite separate diseases, and that the proneness toward depressive disorders in old persons is not due to brain changes of the kind seen in the dementias.

There are four conditions which commonly present difficulties in diagnosis with regard to depressive disorders in the elderly. These are depressive pseudodementia, masked depression, grief reactions, and delusional depression.

Depressive Pseudodementia

Deciding whether an elderly patient suffers from a depression or an early dementia is often a difficult diagnostic task. The two conditions co-exist in a significant number of cases. As many as 25 percent of patients with dementia are depressed. Secondly, and more importantly, depression may mimic organic disease, resulting in mis-diagnosis and therapeutic nihilism rather than proper and effective treatment (See also Chapters 5 and 9.)

Depression is most often mistaken for a progressive dementing process in those cases in which the patient is markedly retarded. This has been described as depressive pseudodementia. Memory defect of variable severity may be elicited on examination along with apathy, neglect of personal appearance, and sometimes even incontinence. In these patients, even careful psychometric investigation may suggest intellectual deterioration.

There are major clinical features differentiating pseudodementia (due to functional psychiatric disorders such as depressive disorders) from 'true' or organic dementia. These features are presented in Table 4.2. Those features which seem most useful in defining depressive pseudodementia are as follows:

1. The onset of depression can be dated. It is usually recent and acute with a relatively short history.
2. Many depressed patients will have a history of previous depressive episodes. There will also be a family history of depressive disorder, often with atypical features.
3. Depressed patients communicate a strong sense of distress. The affect is sustained and more pervasive than in dementia. Depressed patients emphasize disability and highlight their failures.
4. The cognitive impairment in depression is usually not as gross. It is often patchy and inconsistent. Memory loss for recent and remote events is usually equally severe. Demented patients often offer excuses or explanations for failing memory whereas depressed patients are commonly negativistic, refusing to answer or professing overall ignorance ("don't know" answers).
5. The entire picture of depression, including apparent defects in memory, grasp and reasoning, will very often respond dramatically to treatment with antidepressant medication.

One of the most striking features of pseudodemented patients is their marked dependency for both physical care and emotional support. Few patients require such total care as the severely demented, and pseudodemented patients may be striking in the demands they make for care and concern. The use of countertransference feelings may also be helpful in identifying depressive pseudodementia. These patients may make therapists feel sad and many depressive thoughts may come to mind. This is not a charactertistic reaction in dealing with demented patients.

Masked Depression

Elderly patients who are depressed often present with major symptoms in other areas. Somatic complaints, especially pain of unknown origin, are common symptoms of depression. Tiredness, fatigue, and lack of energy are often presenting complaints. Depression may hide behind any alteration in usual behavior. Acting out patterns may involve serious marital disharmony, impulsive sexual behavior, outbursts of rage, and drug and/or alcohol abuse. Cases such as these, where the depressive syndrome is hidden by masking processes such as somatic complaints, fatigue, anger or acting out behavior are described as masked depressions or depressive equivalents. Neither the patient nor the examiner is immediately aware of the underlying mood disorder.

Among elderly patients, somatic masking is very common, and pain is the chief complaint. Once the pain becomes chronic, it is increasingly difficult to distinguish its manifestations and complications from those of depression. For example, patients in chronic pain for any reason typically report loss of appetite,

TABLE 4.2

The Major Clinical Features Differentiating Pseudodementia from Dementia

Pseudodementia	Dementia
Clinical course and history	
Family always aware of dysfunction and its severity	Family often unaware of dysfunction and its severity
Onset can be dated with some precision	Onset can be dated only within broad limits
Symptoms of short duration before medical help is sought	Symptoms usually of long duration before medical help is sought
Rapid progression of symptoms after onset	Slow progression of symptoms throughout course
History of previous psychiatric dysfunction common	History of previous psychiatric dysfunction unusual
Complaints and clinical behaviour	
Patients usually complain much of cognitive loss	Patients usually complain little of cognitive loss
Patients' complaints of cognitive dysfunction usually detailed	Patients' complaints of cognitive dysfunction usually vague
Patients emphasize disability	Patients conceal disability
Patients highlight failures	Patients delight in accomplishments, however trivial
Patients make little effort to perform even simple tasks	Patients struggle to perform tasks
Patients do not try to keep up	Patients rely on notes, calendars, etc., to keep up
Patients usually communicate strong sense of distress	Patients often appear unconcerned
Affective change often pervasive	Affect labile and shallow
Loss of social skills often early and prominent	Social skills often retained
Behavior often incongruent with severity of cognitive dysfunction	Behavior usually compatible with severity of cognitive dysfunction
Nocturnal accentuation of dysfunction uncommon	Nocturnal accentuation of dysfunction common
Clinical features related to memory, cognitive, and intellectual dysfunctions	
Attention and concentration often well preserved	Attention and concentration usually faulty
"Don't know" answers typical	Near-miss answers frequent
On tests of orientation, patients often give "don't know" answers	On tests of orientation, patients often mistake unusual for usual
Memory loss for recent and remote events usually equally severe	Memory loss for recent events usually more severe than for remote events
Memory gaps for specific periods or events common	Memory gaps for specific periods usual*
Marked variability in performance on tasks of similar difficulty	Consistently poor performance on tasks of similar difficulty

*Except when due to delirium, trauma, seizures, etc.

Wells C. E. 1979. "Pseudodementia." *American Journal of Psychiatry.* 136: 895–900.

sleep disturbances, decreased libido, inability to concentrate or to take an interest in things, and loss of ability to function. If questioned directly, these patients will often vigorously deny depression and focus upon the somatic symptom.

The so-called pseudoanergic syndrome is another common form of masked depression. It consists of a wide variety of similar complaints, including loss of energy, fatigue, lassitude, listlessness, languor, weariness, and tiredness. These patients complain of "being all in", "without pep" or "of having no interest". Again, however, there is an absence of a clear description of depressed mood or of other classical features of the depressive syndrome and sadness is typically denied. The masking potential of this picture is enhanced by beliefs of both patients and physicians that decline in energy, listlessness, and easy fatigability are the norm with chronological ageing. In addition, distinguishing fatigue due to organic illness from that due to depression or to mixed organic-depressive states is one of the most difficult tasks in all of medicine.

The treatment of depressive equivalents, once recognized, is identical to that of other depressive syndromes. Antidepressent medication is often highly effective. Further underscoring the importance of diagnosis here is the fact that many patients with masked depressions have suicidal preoccupations by the time they are seen by a psychiatrist.

Although these patients do not report feelings of despair or hopelessness, they may be aware of some of the somatic manifestations of depression such as constipation, loss of appetite, weight loss, or sleep disturbance. In addition, if questioned on how they feel about the masking complaint, they may describe being discouraged and depressed. The complaint itself is usually chronic and careful questioning may reveal diurnal variation, characteristic of the depressive syndrome (i.e., pain worse in the morning than toward evening). These patients have very often suffered at least one episode of depression earlier in life, and they may reveal a family history of depression. And finally, in many cases, history taking should uncover a precipitating event, most often a loss.

Grief

In 1943 Erich Lindemann described the acute grief reaction as a definite syndrome. The five points which establish the diagnosis of grief are outlined in Table 4.3.

TABLE 4.3
Acute Grief Reaction

1.   Somatic distress
2.   Preoccupation with the image of the deceased
3.   Guilt
4.   Hostile reactions
5.   Loss of patterns of conduct

Adapted from Lindemann E. 1944. "Symptomatology and Management of Acute Grief." *American Journal of Psychiatry.* 101: 141.

Grief work is defined as emancipation from bondage to the deceased, re-adjustment to the environment from which the deceased is missing, and the formation of new relationships. If grief work is not accomplished, most often because of avoidance of intense distress connected with the grief experience, then features of inadequate or distorted grief appear. These may include delayed or chronic reactions, overactivity, a recognized medical illness, alteration of relationships with friends and relatives, or a full-blown depressive episode. Therapists, by sharing the patient's grief work in the early stages, can often prevent the development of difficult, distorted reactions. (See also Chapter 2.)

About 20 percent of widowers and widows develop depressive syndromes in the year following the death of the spouse. However, compared to patients with depressive disorder, they have a relative absence of prior episodes of depression and less depressive disorder in their first degree relatives. Also, they have much less tendency to suicidal ideation and they do not define themselves as patients, rather experiencing their distress as a natural reaction to loss.

Factors which delineate persons at high risk for morbid grief reactions include perceived nonsupportiveness in the social network, "traumatic" circumstances of the death, a previously high ambivalent marital relationship and the presence of a concurrent life crisis. Successful resolution of grief correlates with the resumption of social contacts and the development of new interpersonal relations. However, the psychosocial environment of the elderly widow or widower may not provide these crucial substitutions.

Grief reactions in later life may differ. There is a dearth of sadness or conscious guilt. There is less numbness and denial. It is thought that there may be a significant amount of anticipatory grief in elderly people leading to easier acceptance of the loss when it occurs. However, there is a preponderance of somatic illness. Often the onset or accentuation of illness begins at the time of bereavement. Idealization of the image of the deceased is also extreme among elderly mourners and hallucinations and illusions are more common. In contrast to this, there is a tendency toward self-isolation and irrational hostility toward living persons, especially those who may resemble the deceased. Stern (1951) suggests that the most striking feature is the tendency to "channel" material that would produce overt emotional conflict into somatic illness, which may represent self-punishment, a death wish and/or an identification with the deceased.

The importance of recognizing acute grief lies in the opportunity to prevent major complications such as chronic despair and/or disabling dependency by relatively unsophisticated counselling techniques. A series of eight to ten short sessions wherein feelings and memories related to the deceased are ventilated and explored usually suffices. Patients must be brought through acceptance of the loss, adjustment to a world without the spouse and the development of new relationships. In the small percentage of cases who develop late, chronic, full-blown depressive syndromes as complications, treatment should probably be similar to that for depressive disorder. However, this last point requires further research for clarification.

Delusional Depression

Delusional depression refers to depressive disorder in which delusions are the primary manifestation. Thus, delusional depression is characterized by delusional thinking along with other signs of depression. A delusion is a belief held by the patient that can be tested against a known reality, is clearly false, and is not shared by other members of the patient's family or social group. In about 25 percent of cases of delusional depression, patients also experience hallucinations. These hallucinations are nearly always auditory, although visual and kinesthetic hallucinations may occur.

Typically the elderly patient with a delusional depression is very agitated. S/he will have diminished sleep and appetite and will have suffered significant weight loss. S/he will complain of loss of energy, loss of interest in activities, and decreased concentration. S/he will harbor suicidal thoughts and intense feelings of guilt. Examples of delusions include beliefs that the patient will be killed for past transgressions, beliefs that the patient is a criminal as proved by daily news broadcasts, beliefs that a grandchild's injury at camp is the patient's fault, or beliefs that the world is going to end at some preordained time. Auditory hallucinations are most often accusatory. Types of delusions may include guilt, persecution, worthlessness, somatic, hypochondriacal, nihilistic, jealousy, and passivity.

Several features differentiate delusional depression from other depressive disorders. Agitation is much more common in delusional depression whereas other depressed patients tend more often to be anxious and anergic. Delusional depression is also often characterized by ruminations about specific themes, and such patients are markedly self-reproachful. Patients suffering from delusional depression are more likely to have had several prior episodes of depression and these episodes are usually similar in that the same delusion(s) occur each time the patient becomes depressed. Thus, episodes of delusional depression tend to run "true to form." There is a greater frequency of severe family psychiatric disorder, requiring hospitalization, among delusional depressives.

There is also evidence of neurobiological differences between delusional and non-delusional depressives. Delusional depression may be a clinical state mediated by both dopamine and noradrenaline.

Delusional depressed patients respond less well to tricyclic antidepressants than do non-delusional patients. In fact, tricyclics have been shown to exacerbate delusional thinking in these patients when given alone. Antipsychotic medication should be used first to control agitation, sleep difficulties, and delusions. At this point, the patient often becomes dejected with decreased energy and loss of interest in activities, and tricyclic antidepressants are often effective given in combination with the original antipsychotic. Thus, combined drug therapy utilizing antipsychotic and antidepressant medication is the chemotherapeutic treatment of choice. In addition, if chemotherapy fails or is contraindicated, patients with delusional depression are characterized by a very good response to electroconvulsive therapy (ECT). Some clinicians feel that ECT is the treatment of choice for delusional depression.

Diagnostically, delusional depression must be differentiated from other major mental disorders characterized by delusions. These include paranoid schizophrenia, schizoaffective disorders, paranoid disorders, and acute and chronic organic brain disorders.

Paranoid schizophrenia and schizoaffective disorders present with non-affective psychotic signs and symptoms in addition to delusions and hallucinations. These may include flattened affect, loosened associations, autistic withdrawal, thought broadcasting, thought control, thought withdrawal and insertion, and other well-known features of schizophrenic disorders. Patients with delusional depression do not demonstrate the characteristic formal thought disorder seen in schizophrenia and schizoaffective disorders.

Paranoid disorders resemble delusional depression most closely. However, patients with paranoid disorders do not present with other features of the depressive syndrome. In addition, patients with depressive disorders tend to have obsessive and/or dependent traits in their premorbid personality whereas paranoid patients have paranoid and narcissistic personality features. Most importantly, underlying depressive delusions are feelings of intense guilt and self-reproach related to the core depressive affect. Thus, whatever the false belief, the patient feels deserving of punishment. The affect underlying delusions in paranoid disorders, on the other hand, is usually hostility. The patient is frequently enraged at the injustice inherent in his/her delusional perceptions of the world and acting out, when it occurs, tends to be other-directed rather than self-directed as in depressive states.

Delusions in organic brain syndromes tend not to be as fully-formed as in delusional depressions. In dementias, delusions are accompanied by signs of intellectual deterioration and cognitive deficits. In confusional states, delusions are accompanied by clouding of consciousness and hallucinations are frequently visual. Affect is more often fearful than depressed. It should be noted that some patients with delusional depression may appear to present cognitive deficits (pseudodementia). However, these deficits do respond to treatment with combined drug therapy or ECT. Finally, a history of previous episodes of delusional depression often helps in differential diagnosis, as does a family history of depressive disorder.

SUICIDE

As mentioned above, the elderly account for an inordinately high proportion of suicides. Most elderly suicides are mentally ill, predominantly with a depressive disorder, usually their first. The risk of suicide for the elderly depressive is many times that for the younger depressive, and four times greater for male depressives than for females. Physical illness is a far more important risk factor for the older than the younger suicide.

In a series of 30 suicides over age 65, a history of insomnia, weight loss, and reduction in activities was found in nearly all cases. Two-thirds had been depressed less than one year. One week after seeing their general practitioner just under half died, and 90 percent had seen him/her within the previous three months. Only five had been prescribed antidepressants, but in three instances not in adequate doses. Only two had been referred to a psychiatrist.

This study also revealed a clear excess of physical illness among the suicides. In most cases (87 percent), some form of depressive syndrome was present and its onset appeared to have been in relation to the onset of the physical illness.

In almost every study, living alone is a factor related to increased suicide risk in the elderly. Anniversaries of significant bereavements, especially of a father's death, may influence an old person's suicide.

The elderly person at high risk for suicide is typically a male suffering from a depressive disorder who has lost one of his parents in childhood from suicide, and who has himself threatened or attempted suicide. He will be living alone, may have been recently discharged from hospital, and will have experienced recent bereavement or physical illness. He may also be drinking heavily.

Prevention depends upon a number of factors. One is the recognition of the potentially lethal combination of age and severe depression, especially in the presence of physical illness. Most suicides give a clear warning, more often than not to a physician. It thus behooves us to recognize the warning and to act effectively. Treatment of depressive disorders must be thorough with aggressive follow-up. Half-treated depressives may have an even higher suicidal risk. Elderly depressed patients who do not respond to treatment should be referred to psychiatrists. In addition, improvement of the elderly patients' physical health so that minor ailments which limit their well-being and mobility are eradicated or at least ameliorated, is an important suicide prevention measure. (See also Chapter 9.)

CAUSES

Biology

It now appears that some depressive disorders are genetically determined. It has also been reported that depression appearing at a later age may be genetically different from early onset forms. In fact, it is generally accepted that there is an inverse relationship between age at first attack of depression and strength of genetic factors. Patients who develop depression for the first time in old age have much less depressive disorder in their families. This has led to the assumption that physiological, psychological, or psychosocial precipitants might be of greater significance than in younger depressives. The risk factor in first degree relatives of depressive patients with an age of onset above 50 is about 8 percent compared to 20 percent for the relatives of patients with an age of onset below 50. Late onset probably indicates a smaller genetic and correspondingly greater environmental component. This "environmental component" usually refers to psychological events which are stressful.

With regard to biochemical causes or changes in depression, the biogenic amine hypothesis suggests that depression is associated with alterations in the synthesis, storage, release, and utilization of chemical neurotransmitters. Enzymes involved in these mechanisms are thought to be under genetic control. Thus deficiencies of catecholamines and/or indoleamines at functionally important receptor sites in the brain have been thought to be associated with depression. (See also Chapter 11.)

Monoamine oxidase (MAO) is an enzyme responsible for the inactivation of several biogenic amines in the central nervous system. It has been found in higher concentrations in both platelets and plasma of depressed patients. In one group of patients, the administration of oral conjugated estrogen decreased plasma MAO and improved mood. Thus the increasing levels of MAO activity that occur with normal ageing, along with alterations in gonadal function in the elderly may relate to the higher incidence of depression via diminution of functional amines at synaptic junctions.

A relationship between both decreased thyroid function and decreased hypothalamic releasing hormone and depression has been suggested. This may give some significance to the diminishing thyroid function and the diminishing responsiveness of the pituitary to hypothalamic thyroid releasing factor that occurs with ageing.

Finally, several biochemical changes more frequently seen in late onset than in early onset depressions have been identified. These are increased 3-methoxy-4-hydroxy-phenyl-glycol (a metabolite of norepinephrine) concentrations in the urine, decreased testosterone and/or estrogen levels in the serum, and increased MAO activity in plasma, platelets, and human hindbrain. However, as Lipton states, it would appear at present that "there are really very little data on the biology of depression which are not controversial and even less on the biology of ageing as it relates to depression" (1976, 5).

Loss

Old age has been described as a season of loss, and depressions have often been understood psychodynamically as excessive responses to losses, either real or imagined. Physical decline results in degrees of impairment of special senses, and chronic illnesses produce discomfort and loss of stamina, vigor and mobility. Flexible intelligence diminishes with age, so-called benign amnesia develops and reaction time is slowed. Most important are psychosocial changes. Retirement precipitates role and income loss. The loss of friends through death contributes to growing social isolation and loneliness. Loss of spouse through death produces grief and through separation/divorce may stimulate rage and hostility. Awareness of one's own impending mortality may follow from any of the physical or psychosocial losses mentioned above.

Depressive disorders in many elderly persons are precipitated by physical or psychological stresses. This was found to be the case in 60 percent of consecutive patients in one series and in 70 to 80 percent in a later investigation. These precipitating events, which could be interpreted in almost all instances as presenting one form or other of "loss", were of a kind commonly borne by all ageing persons. In one series, physical illness, interpreted as threatened loss, had preceded depression in 24 percent and psychological or social losses were connected with the depression in 36 percent. It has been suggested that older people can tolerate the loss of loved objects and of prestige better than a decline in physical health. In the category of losses, it has also been shown that elderly depressives have an increased prevalence of loss of a parent in childhood, which event is thought to confer increased vulnerability to depressive disorder.

A very extensive and careful study investigated the relationship of both past and current losses to depression. It established that recent events with long-term threatening implications, most of which involved some major loss, play a significant role in bringing about depressive disorders. In addition, certain kinds of long-term difficulties appear to play a causal but less important role. With regard to past losses, loss of a mother before age 11 is associated with greater risk of depression, and all types of past loss by death correlate with severity of depressive symptoms. Among a sample of depressed women, those who were 50 to 65 were much more likely to have experienced past loss than those aged 20 to 35. This may help explain the increased prevalence of severe depression among the elderly.

Depression in the aged has been described as predominantly due to a "recognition of weakness and an inability to obtain necessary narcissistic supplies or defend against threats to security" (Busse 1955, 901). Thus the old person's losses undermine security and attacks ongoing self-esteem. This produces a sense of helplessness and powerlessness which has been identified as the core dynamic in depression at any age. Thus grief and/or guilt may be less important in reacting to the losses with ageing, but rather profound hopelessness about one's ability to control the world, to repair damage, and to obtain alternative sources of value may predominate. This may also explain the increased vulnerability of people who have suffered early object loss. Until a child is about 11, his/her main means of controlling the world is likely to be his/her mother. The earlier she is lost, the more the child is likely to be set back in his/her learning of mastery of the environment, and this sense of mastery is an essential component of self-esteem. Thus, the combination of lifelong impaired self-esteem with the deprivation of important sources of value in old age may result in a profound sense of helplessness, hopelessness, and powerlessness which colors the depressive disorders in the elderly.

MANAGEMENT

Treatment of the elderly patient with a depressive syndrome which meets the criteria of a major depressive disorder should be as aggressive as possible. Tricyclic antidepressants, monoamine oxidase inhibitors, lithium carbonate, and electroconvulsive therapy are the mainstays. The efficacy of some "second generation" antidepressants has been claimed for the elderly, but remains to be demonstrated. Supportive psychotherapy in severe to moderate depression and exploratory psychotherapy in mild depression are also indicated, sometimes in conjunction with benzodiazepines or antidepressants.

Special concerns involved in antidepressant drug treatment of the elderly include: a) alterations in absorption, distribution, metabolism, detoxification, and excretion of drugs; b) increased vulnerability to adverse side effects; c) adjustment of dosage downward to achieve therapeutic effects without undue hazard of toxicity; d) interaction with other drugs used in treatment of concomitant physical illnesses; and, e) complications introduced by acute or chronic physical diseases. (See also Chapter 11.)

Tricyclic compounds should be the initial pharmacological approach to depressive disorders. These drugs block the re-uptake of norepinephrine by adrenergic nerve terminals. The demethylated analogs such as desipramine are more potent in this action, whereas the methylated drugs such as imipramine and amitriptyline are more potent in the blockade of serotonin re-uptake. Although the exact relationship of these effects to the actions of the tricyclic antidepressants in humans is not known, they have contributed significantly to the "biogenic amine hypothesis" of depression. Major reviews should be consulted for further information.

Tricyclic antidepressants should never be prescribed on an "as-needed" basis. The relatively slow onset of action probably relates to changes in biogenic amine metabolism. If these drugs are given over a period of time to depressed patients, an elevation of mood occurs, usually after two to three weeks.

There is disagreement as to whether tricyclic dosages should be reduced in elderly patients. It has been shown however, that older depressed patients do develop higher steady-state plasma levels associated with a decreased rate of drug elimination from plasma. These findings may explain the increased susceptibility to tricyclic side effects in older patients. However, the relationship of plasma levels to therapeutic efficacy is not yet clear.

Tricyclic side effects of particular importance in the elderly include anticholinergic, neurologic, and cardiovascular problems. Urinary retention may be an especially difficult complication in elderly males. Toxic encephalopathies presenting as confusional syndromes are much more common in older patients. Cardiovascular side effects are potentially the most dangerous complication of tricyclic treatment and so low doses, small spaced increases, careful monitoring of vital signs, and serial ECG's are strongly indicated in elderly patients with pre-existing cardiovascular disease. (See also Chapter 11.)

The treatment of depression in medically ill geriatric patients is feasible using antidepressant medication. However, the presence of multisystem disease can appear to be an insurmountable obstacle. In particular, cardiovascular and pulmonary diseases require caution. Orthostatic hypotension, tachyarrhythmias, and congestive heart failure are dangerous complications. In addition, tricyclics have mild respiratory depressant effects at therapeutic doses. There is no question that in these patients, very low initial dosages with careful monitoring of small increases is essential.

Finally, it is useful to know that predictors of good response to tricyclic antidepressants in all age groups include insidious onset, anorexia, weight loss, middle and late insomnia, and psychomotor disturbance. Predictors of poor response are neurotic hypochondriacal and hysterical traits, multiple prior episodes, and delusions.

The monoamine oxidase inhibitors (MAOI) present a second line of pharmacological attack on the depressive syndrome. They are thought to be most useful when atypical symptoms occur such as hypochondriasis, anxiety, irritability, phobias, and/or anergia. MAO inhibition increases brain dopamine, norepinephrine, and serotonin. Recent work has suggested that in order to be effective these drugs must be given in doses high enough to produce a significant degree of enzyme inhibition. Such doses may often need to be higher than were previously recommended (i.e., phenelzine 60 mg. daily). As with the tricyclics, these drugs do not produce benefits immediately. The time between first administration of the drug and clinical response may vary from several days to a few weeks.

With monoamine oxidase inhibitors (MAOI), hypertensive crises are extremely rare when patients are given dietary instructions. Orthostatic hypotension is a much more common and troublesome side effect in the elderly, and dosage reduction may be necessary to maintain blood pressure. These drugs have a psychostimulating effect and so may produce insomnia and increased anxiety in some patients. On the other hand, this effect may be advantageous in the apathetic, depressed elderly patient.

Regarding drug interactions, antacids block gastrointestinal absorption and so decrease antidepressant drug levels, as do barbiturates which should not be prescribed for the elderly. Phenothiazines increase serum levels and may enhance therapeutic response. Tricyclics may antagonize the B-receptor blocking and antiarrhythmic action of propanalol as well as interfere with the therapeutic action of anticoagulants. Furthermore, tricyclics may interfere with the antihypertensive effect of alpha-methyldopa and inhibit the antihypertensive action of guanethidine and its cogeners.

With regard to lithium, the need for lower daily doses to achieve adequate blood levels relates to the longer half-life of lithium in the elderly. This is because of the significant decrease in renal glomerular filtration with age. Both therapeutic and toxic effects occur at much lower dosage and serum levels than in younger persons. Lithium doses under 900 mg. daily and blood levels under 1.0 m Eq/litre are recommended.

Old age is not a contraindication to electroconvulsive therapy. When the depressive syndrome is very severe or life-threatening or when an adequate trial of antidepressant medication has failed, then ECT should be considered. In fact, it may be safer than many psychotropic drugs because it does not have their many side effects.

Careful cardiovascular investigation is necessary before an elderly person is placed on ECT. Patients with recent myocardial infarctions or decompensated heart failure should probably be excluded. No essential change in technique is necessary. However, treatments should be spaced further apart, so that the number of ECT's should be kept to a minimum. Premature interruption may lead to relapse. If post-ECT confusion is severe, then frequency of treatments should be further diminished. A usual course includes eight to ten treatments given over five to six weeks. Factors associated with good response to ECT include family history of depression, early morning awakening, delusions, and psychomotor retardation. (See also Chapter 11.)

Less severe depressions respond mainly to psychotherapy. A particular approach to brief therapy with such patients has been described. As the elderly patient's conviction of helplessness and ineffectuality develops in response to losses and the absence of substitute gratifications, s/he seeks a powerful, protective figure, often a physician, to help restore feelings of security. Thus, as the patient becomes convinced of good standing with the therapist, the individual's self-esteem is increased. As Goldfarb suggests, "the feeling of worth grows out of the relationship nurtured by the therapist. As his (patient's) self-regard mounts his sense of helplessness decreases" (1953, 918).

Countertransference, which is the emotional reactions of the therapist to the patient, is a major obstacle to psychotherapy with elderly patients. Especially with the depressed patient, anxiety is aroused in the therapist by the unconscious identification with the patient's helplessness. In addition, discomfort is often aroused in dealing with the sexual problems of the aged. Also, it is important to understand the so-called "reversed transference"—the tendency of the older patient to view the therapist as his/her child. This relationship must be allowed to develop, as it offers the patient an opportunity to rework fundamental relationships. Thus, the good son- or daughter-therapist should not feel guilty for being younger. The older patient will often attempt to elicit such guilt and anxiety as a defence against working through important conflicts.

In keeping with his/her formulation of depression as a result of a sense of helplessness and powerlessness, Bibring (1953) outlined ways in which depression may be resolved. These are often helpful in dealing psychotherapeutically with the elderly patient as they may become goals in short-term therapy. They include:

1. When a goal which seemed unreachable again appears within reach.
2. When the goal is sufficiently modified to become reachable.
3. When the goal is abandoned.
4. When self-esteem is recovered through other means, with or without change in the unreachable goal.
5. When a defence is erected against the depressing feeling (Bibring 1953, 126).

Within a supportive relationship which contains aspects of earlier important relationships and which itself may enhance self-esteem, depressed elderly patients may work toward one or more of these methods of resolution of depression.

REFERENCES AND SUGGESTED READINGS

American Psychiatric Association. 1980. *Diagnostic and Statistical Manual of Mental Disorders.* 3rd ed.

Ban T. A. 1978. "The Treatment of Depressed Geriatric Patients." *American Journal of Psychotherapy.* 32: 1.

Barraclough B. 1972. "Suicide in the Elderly." *Recent Developments in Psychogeriatrics.* Ed. D. Kay and A. Walk. British Journal of Psychiatry Special Publication No. 6.

Bielski R. J. and R. O. Friedel. 1976. "Prediction of Tricyclic Antidepressant Response." *Archives of General Psychiatry.* 37: 1479.

Bibring E. 1953. "The Mechanism of Depression." *Affective Disorders.* Ed. P. Greenacre. New York: International Universities Press.

Briscoe C. and J. Smith. 1975. "Depression in Bereavement and Divorce." *Archives of General Psychiatry.* 32: 439.

Brown G. W., T. Harris and J. R. Copeland. 1977. "Depression and Loss." *British Journal of Psychiatry.* 130: 1.

Brown R. P. and J. H. Koesis et al. 1984. "Efficacy and Feasibility of High Dose Tricyclic Antidepressant Treatment in Elderly Delusional Depressives." *Journal of Clinical Psychopharmacology.* 9: 311.

Busse E. W., R. H. Barnes and A. J. Silverman. 1955. "Studies of the Process of Aging. The Strengths and Weaknesses of Psychic Functioning in the Aged." *American Journal of Psychiatry.* 111: 896.

Carlson R. S. 1976. "Pre-senile Dementia Presenting As A Depressive Illness." *Canadian Psychiatric Association Journal.* 21: 527.

Cavenar J. O., A. A. Maltbie and L. Austin. 1979. "Depression Simulating Organic Brain Disease." *American Journal of Psychiatry.* 136: 521.

Davis J. M. 1973. "Theories of Biological Etiology of Affective Disorders." *International Review of Neurobiology.* 12: 145.

Dovenmuehle R. H. and A. Verwoerdt. 1962. "Physical Illness and Depressive Symptomatology." *Journal of American Geriatric Society.* 10: 932.

Dunn C. G. and D. Gross. "Treatment of Depression in the Medically Ill Geriatric Patient: A Case Report." *American Journal of Psychiatry.* 134: 4.

Eastwood R. 1978. "Prevention of Suicide." *Preventive Medicine and Public Health.* Ed. J. Last. New York: Appleton-Century-Crofts.

Epstein L. J. 1976. "Depression in the Elderly." *Journal of Gerontology.* 31: 3.

Foster J. R., W. J. Gershell and A. J. Goldfarb. 1977. "Lithium Treatment in the Elderly." *Journal of Gerontology.* 32: 3.

Goldfarb A. and H. Turner. 1953. "Psychotherapy and Aged Persons II. Utilization and Effectiveness of 'Brief' Therapy." *American Journal of Psychiatry.* 109: 916.

Goodman L. S. and A. Gilman. 1975. *The Pharmacological Basis of Therapeutics.* 5th ed. New York: MacMillan Publishing Co. Inc.

Grotjohn M. 1955. "Analytic Psychotherapy with the Elderly." *Psychoanalytic Review.* 42: 419.

Gurland B. J. 1976. "The Comparative Frequency of Depression in Various Adult Age Groups." *Journal of Gerontology.* 31: 3.

Karno M. and R. Hoffman. 1974. "The Pseudoanergic Syndrome." *Somatic Manifestations of Depressive Disorders.* Ed. A. Kiev. Excerpta Medica.

Kral V. A. December 1972. "Depressions in the Aged and Their Treatment." *Psychiatry Digest.* 49.

Kral V. A. 1976. "Somatic Therapies in Older Depressed Patients." *Journal of Gerontology.* 31: 3.

Lesse S. 1967. "Hypochondriasis and Psychosomatic Disorders Masking Depression." *American Journal of Psychotherapy.* 21: 607.

Lindemann E. 1944. "Symptomatology and Management of Acute Grief." *American Journal of Psychiatry.* 101: 141.

Lipton M. 1976. "Age Differentiation in Depression: Biochemical Aspects." *Journal of Gerontology.* 31: 3.

Mendels J. 1965. "Electroconvulsive Therapy and Depression." *British Journal of Psychiatry.* 111: 687.

Mendlewicz J. 1976. "The Age Factor in Depressive Illness: Some Genetic Considerations." *Journal of Gerontology.* 31: 3.

Nelson J. C. and M. B. Bowers. 1978. "Delusional Unipolar Depression." *Archives of General Psychiatry.* 35: 1321.

Nies A. 1977. "Relationship Between Age and Tricyclic Antidepressant Plasma Levels." *American Journal of Psychiatry.* 134: 7.

Pfeiffer E. and E. Busse. 1973. "Mental Disorders in Later Life—Affective Disorders, Paranoid, Neurotic and Situational Reactions." *Mental Illness in Later Life.* Ed. E. Busse and E. Pfeiffer. Washington: American Psychiatric Association.

Stern K., G. M. Williams and M. Prados. 1951. "Grief Reactions in Later Life." *American Journal of Psychiatry.* 108: 289.

Weissman M. M. and J. K. Myers. 1979. "Depression in the Elderly: Research Directions of Psychopathology, Epidemiology and Treatment." *Journal of Geriatric Psychiatry.* 12: 187.

Wells C. E. 1979. "Pseudodementia." *American Journal of Psychiatry.* 136: 895.

5

Dementia

Barry A. Martin, M.D., F.R.C.P. (C)

The most appropriate paradigm or unifying concept for both the normal and pathological sequelae of ageing is that of "loss". The net effect of ageing, in varying degrees, is an accumulation of physical and psychological losses. There is a progressive decline in physical integrity through normal wear and tear, the acquisition of chronic degenerative diseases, and often an increased susceptibility to acute illness. The psychological losses encountered when growing old are protean. They may be brought about by the geographic separation from and deaths of relatives and friends and by changes in social roles. These untoward sequelae of the ageing process have been summarized rather poignantly by William Shakespeare in Act II, Scene VII of *As You Like It*:

> All the world's a stage, and all the men and women merely players:
> They have their exits and their entrances; And one man in his
> time plays many parts, his acts being seven ages ... Last scene
> of all, that ends this strange eventful history, is second childishness
> and mere oblivion, sans teeth, sans eyes, sans taste, sans everything.

Turning to the field of geriatric psychiatry, the same paradigm applies since a number of mental disorders may be caused or precipitated by or associated with the above-noted physical, psychological, and social losses. The most important of these disorders, in terms of numbers affected, is depression as described in the preceding chapter. Real or imagined losses, the loss of self-esteem, or the loss of the ability to achieve an idealized self-image are some of the unifying psychodynamic concepts for depression. This chapter addresses one of the most serious physical losses that occurs with ageing, the loss of neurons in the brain, and the mental disorder caused by that loss, dementia.

The human brain consists of approximately 100 billion neurons or nerve cells, about the same number as stars in our galaxy. Neurons are the anatomic elements of the information transmission network of the brain, each cell having approximately 1 000 to 10 000 synapses or connections with other neurons.

There is an enormous reserve capacity of the brain such that many cells may be lost without noticeable impairment, particularly if those lost cells are distributed widely throughout the brain or are involved in brain functions that are not readily apparent during daily activities. However, if there is a concentration of neuronal loss in one part of the brain or the loss of too many neurons serving a highly visible brain function, for example memory or language, the consequent impairment or disability may be substantial. In order to understand the clinical presentation and course of dementia, the overall distribution and quantity of nerve cell loss in the brain must be appreciated.

DEFINITION

Dementia is a syndrome or group of symptoms with diverse causes and a variable course. The specific symptoms of dementia result from the structural loss or death of nerve cells which subserve specific integrative or cognitive functions of the brain (see Clinical Features). Although cases with an acute onset and static or non-progressive course are often subsumed under the term "dementia", its usual connotation is that of the insidious onset of global cognitive impairment which is progressive as long as the pathogenesis or disease process remains uninterrupted. If detected early enough, the syndrome may be partially or completely reversible if the etiology or cause is known and the pathogenesis can be altered by specific treatment. The death of very large numbers of nerve cells results in the gross atrophy of the overall brain mass.

CLASSIFICATION

As previously noted, dementia is a syndrome in that a number of disease processes may lead to progressive global, cognitive impairment. While a specific cause of the syndrome may be demonstrable, reviews of cases assessed at neurological centres indicate that more than 50 percent are idiopathic or of unknown cause and almost all of these are now thought to be cases of Alzheimer's disease. (In nursing homes and psychiatric facilities, a much higher proportion of the demented patients have Alzheimer's disease since other cases are treated and/or referred elsewhere.) Although once considered a disease with its onset in the presenium, the pathology in the brains of patients with an onset after age 65 is not distinct. Therefore, all cases are grouped together in the latest classification as primary degenerative dementia, Alzheimer type, with the age of onset classified secondarily. Parenthetically, the designation of age 65 as the onset of senescence has no biological basis; in particular, there are no changes in the brain which uniformly begin at that point in the course of normal ageing.

In the past, many cases of dementia were thought to be caused by cerebral arteriosclerosis. However, at autopsy, very little correlation has been found between the degree of narrowing of the cerebral arteries and the degree of cognitive impairment before death. Many patients with severe cerebral arteriosclerosis exhibit no evidence of dementia while others with little vascular disease are severely demented. Most of these patients are now classified as cases of Alzheimer's disease. When the dementia is caused by a series of strokes (cerebrovascular accidents), it is now classified as multi-infarct dementia.

The relative numerical importance of many of the disorders that may present clinically with symptoms of dementia is summarized in Table 5.1. These are the diagnoses in three series of cases investigated for the cause of dementia at neurological centres. Unfortunately, there is no specific treatment that will either halt the progress of or substantially reverse the cognitive impairment found in the great majority of patients in these diagnostic groups. However, medical or surgical treatment of the underlying condition may result in the complete reversal of the dementia in a small proportion, perhaps 10 to 15 percent, if detected early enough. Therefore, it is axiomatic that all cases of recent onset be investigated thoroughly for a treatable cause. The clinical investigation protocol suggested in Table 5.2 includes various tests to detect many of the disorders noted in Table 5.1

TABLE 5.1

Diagnoses of Patients with Symptoms of Dementia

Diagnosis	Number of Patients	Percentage of Caseload
Atrophy of unknown cause (Alzheimer's disease)	113	51
Vascular disease (including multi-infarct dementia)	17	8
Normal pressure hydrocephalus	14	6
Dementia in alcoholics (including Korsakoff's syndrome)	13	6
Intracranial masses	12	5
Huntington's disease	10	5
Depression	9	4
Drug toxicity	7	3
Dementia (uncertain)	7	3
Other disorders[1]	20	9

[1]Each accounting for less than 1 percent of the caseload: Creutzfeldt-Jakob disease, post-traumatic, thyroid disease, post-encephalitic, other psychiatric disorders, neurosyphilis, amyotrophic lateral sclerosis, post-subarachnoid hemorrhage, Parkinson's disease, pernicious anemia, liver failure, epilepsy.

Adapted from Wells C. E. 1978. "Chronic Brain Disease: An Overview." *American Journal of Psychiatry.* 135: 1–12.

It should be noted that some functional mental disorders may present with symptoms of dementia. This can be a difficult differential diagnosis to resolve so that a complete mental status examination is necessary. (See also Chapter 4 and Chapter 9.) On careful examination, it is found that there is no cognitive impairment and, of course, there is no neuronal loss underlying the symptoms in such cases. Therefore, they are more accurately referred to as cases of pseudodementia. This is not a separate diagnostic classification since all cases, when correctly identified, are placed in other diagnostic groups, usually depression.

TABLE 5.2
Clinical Investigation of Dementia[1]

1. History
2. General physical examination
3. Complete neurological examination
4. Complete mental status examination
5. CT scan
6. Haemoglobin and erythrocyte indexes
7. Leukocyte count and differential
8. Serum B_{12}
9. Thyroid function screening: T_3 and T_4
10. Hepatic and renal function screening
11. Drug screening
12. Serum glucose: 2-hour p.c.
13. Serology for syphilis: VDRL
14. EEG
15. EKG

[1]A CT scan is the single most useful investigation to confirm the presence of significant atrophy, either focal or generalized, and/or intracranial masses. The remaining tests are suggested as a general screening for diseases that may cause or contribute to impaired cognitive function. The clinical indications for some individual tests are determined, in part, by the history and the findings on physical examination.

FREQUENCY AND DISTRIBUTION

In Canada, the life expectancy of males is now over 71 years and that for females is over 78 years. Those 65 years of age now constitute about 9 percent of the total population. That proportion is steadily increasing so that by the end of the century it may be approximately 13 percent.

When the results of a number of studies are considered, it may be estimated that 5 percent of the population over 65 years of age has severe dementia and a further 5 percent has milder forms. The point prevalence (number of cases in the population at any given point in time) increases with age, particularly after age 75. In every age group over 65, females have higher prevalence rates than males because of their greater life expectancy. Since those over age 65 constitute about 10 percent of the population, approximately one percent of the total population has dementia. It is very difficult to determine the true incidence of dementia (the number of new cases) but a crude estimate may be an annual rate of one percent of the population over age 65. There is no evidence that the incidence rate is increasing.

The prevalence of dementia is increasing, primarily the result of earlier case detection and an increased life expectancy after the onset of illness. Thus, as opposed to findings in the 1950's that most patients died within one or two years, lifespan after disease detection today is in the order of four to eight years. (These figures refer to patients who would now be diagnosed as having Alzheimer's disease.) Since the life expectancy of the general population has been quite static over this period, the increased survivorship of those with dementia is probably the result of more effective medical management of intercurrent disease. Of course, this increases the burden upon those who must care for the dementing patients since the mental status deteriorates over time. Even the caseload that is institutionalized late in the course of the illness has a substantial survivorship. For example, review of the death and discharge log books for the years 1969 to 1978 at one nursing home, admitting mostly demented patients from the Toronto area, revealed that from the time of admission, 50 percent of residents were dead after two years and 70 percent after four years.

Apart from age and sex, no other demographic correlations with a diagnosis of Alzheimer's disease are known. There are no demographic factors, for example premorbid education or socio-economic status, which protect against developing the disease. While there is some evidence for a familial clustering of cases and a possible genetic causal factor, most patients have no family history of dementia. Patients with Down's syndrome have a higher incidence of Alzheimer's disease than the general population.

PATHOLOGICAL CHANGES IN THE BRAIN

In conceptualizing the pathological changes that occur in Alzheimer's disease, it is useful to consider their relationship to those that occur with normal ageing. Normal ageing is associated with declining mental acuity. This is primarily the result of a slowing of thought processes, rather than absolute loss, and mild forgetfulness which has been designated "benign senescence". While there are very limited normative data for the elderly, there is relatively little decline in verbal intelligence on formal testing. In addition, if given sufficient time, there is little decline in non-verbal or performance intelligence. Nevertheless, the declining intellectual acuity is associated with anatomical changes in the brain.

As previously noted, the human brain consists of approximately 100 billion neurons, all present from birth. The brain reaches its maximum weight at about 20 years. Thereafter, the population of neurons decreases, with the loss most concentrated in the frontal and temporal lobes of the brain. (The location of the lobes of the cortex of the brain is depicted in Figure 5.1.)

In neuropathological terminology, the anatomical changes that are found as neurons die with age are intraneuronal neurofibrillary tangles, senile plaques, and granulovacuolar degeneration. These are indistinguishable from those which occur in Alzheimer's disease. At autopsy, it is found that the incidence of these changes in "normal" brains increases with age so that by age 70 all are affected. Thus, pathologically, the normal ageing brain and that of Alzheimer's disease seem to differ only quantitatively. With the onset of Alzheimer's disease, the rate of neuronal loss increases. In addition, there is further concentration of that loss in the frontal and temporal lobes and the hippocampal formation, part of the brain which is necessary for incorporating new learning into memory.

Again, it is important to correlate the degree and concentration of neuronal loss with specific symptoms. The gross anatomy of the lobes of the cerebral cortex is illustrated in Figure 5.1. Several of the cognitive functions predominantly subserved by each of the lobes are noted. These functions are not confined entirely to the specific lobes since there is considerable functional interaction among contiguous cortical areas. For example, the understanding and expression of speech involves functions mediated by the frontal, parietal, and temporal lobes as illustrated. The diagram depicts a lateral view of the surface of the brain. The hippocampal gyrus of the temporal lobe which is required for the formation of new memories lies on the mesial or inside surface of the cortex.

FIGURE 5.1

The Cerebral Cortex of the Human Brain: Localization of Cognitive Functions

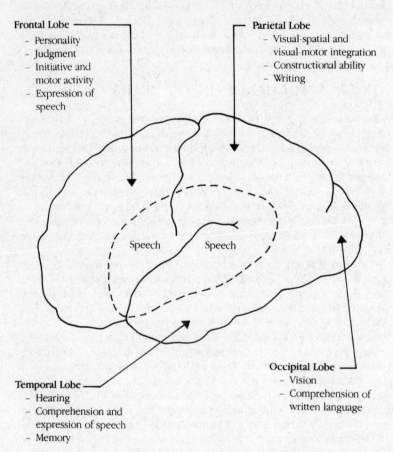

Frontal Lobe
- Personality
- Judgment
- Initiative and motor activity
- Expression of speech

Parietal Lobe
- Visual-spatial and visual-motor integration
- Constructional ability
- Writing

Speech   Speech

Temporal Lobe
- Hearing
- Comprehension and expression of speech
- Memory

Occipital Lobe
- Vision
- Comprehension of written language

Some cognitive functions (i.e. speech and language, visual-motor organization) require the very complex integration of large cortical areas. Others, such as the formation of new memories, require relatively small areas. The various symptoms and behavioral changes of dementia described in the next section are the results of neuronal loss in the areas of the brain subserving the previously mentioned functions. Some symptoms require an extensive loss of neurons before they become readily apparent. On the other hand, a relatively small amount of cell loss in strategic locations in the brain may be associated with very gross functional impairment. In these instances, quite profound dementia may occur in the presence of very little overall atrophy of the brain mass. Therefore, on gross examination, such as by CT scan, the brain may appear normal for the patient's age.

CLINICAL FEATURES

The clinical presentations of dementia are extremely diverse depending upon the areas of the brain most involved in the disease process at any given time. Therefore, the diagnosis may not be readily apparent. Many studies attest to the fact that the syndrome is over- and under-diagnosed in a large proportion of cases. Unfortunately, an erroneous diagnosis may have substantive implications for the patient. Therefore, it has been essential to define minimum criteria which must be met before the diagnosis can be made with any certainty.

TABLE 5.3

DSM—III Diagnostic Criteria

Dementia

A. A loss of intellectual abilities of sufficient severity to interfere with social or occupational functioning.

B. Memory impairment.

C. At least one of the following:
1. impairment of abstract thinking
2. impaired judgment
3. other disturbances of higher cortical function, such as aphasia, apraxia, agnosia, constructional apraxia
4. personality change

D. State of consciousness not clouded (i.e. does not meet the criteria for delirium or intoxication, although these may be superimposed).

E. Either 1 or 2:
1. evidence from the history, physical examination, or laboratory tests, of a specific organic factor that is judged to be etiologically related to the disturbance.
2. in the absence of such evidence, an organic factor necessary for the development of the syndrome can be presumed if conditions other than organic mental disorders have been reasonably excluded and if the behavioral change represents cognitive impairment in a variety of areas.

The diagnostic criteria for dementia have been specified most clearly in the *Diagnostic and Statistical Manual of Mental Disorders, Third Edition* (DSM-III) and they are summarized in Table 5.3. In keeping with World Health Organization concepts of case definition in psychiatry, the intellectual loss must exceed a certain threshold of severity to produce some social disability. Impairment of the ability to acquire new memories is central to the syndrome, and, in particular, to Alzheimer's disease as described later. The diffuse distribution of neuronal loss is evidenced by disturbance of one or more other cognitive or integrative functions of the cerebral cortex. As a result of impaired abstract reasoning, thinking becomes concrete with a loss of creativity. Social judgment is impaired, often with disinhibition. Other more specific cognitive losses may include: aphasia, the inability to comprehend or express speech; agnosia, the inability to recognize various stimuli when the primary sensory modalities (i.e. touch) remain intact; and, apraxia and impaired constructional ability, the inability to perform previously learned or complex integrated motor tasks. The personality changes that may occur are described below. The level of consciousness is normal as opposed to that in delirium or toxic syndromes. A specific organic cause may be found or presumed if the functional mental disorders have been ruled out in the presence of global cognitive impairment.

TABLE 5.4

DSM—III   Diagnostic Criteria

Primary Degenerative Dementia—Alzheimer Type

A. Dementia
B. Insidious onset with uniformly progresssive deteriorating course.
C. Exclusion of all other specific causes of dementia by the history, physical examination and laboratory tests.

Multi-Infarct Dementia

A. Dementia
B. Stepwise deteriorating course (not uniformly progressive) with "patchy" distribution of deficits (affecting some functions, but not others) early in the course.
C. Focal neurological signs and symptoms (exaggeration of deep tendon reflexes, extensor plantar response, pseudobulbar palsy, gait abnormalities, weakness of an extremity, etc.,).
D. Evidence, from the history, physical examination, or laboratory tests, of significant cerebrovascular disease that is judged to be etiologically related to the disturbance.

American Psychiatric Association Diagnostic and Statistical Manual of Mental Disorders, Third Edition. Washington, DC, copyright APA 1980. Used with permission.

The diagnostic criteria for Alzheimer's disease and multi-infarct dementia are summarized in Table 5.4. Both require the above-noted criteria for dementia. Alzheimer's disease is invariably insidious in onset even though stressful events may precipitate sudden deterioration. On closer history, it is found that such events have just unmasked a tenuous equilibrium maintained by the patient early in the course of illness and the onset can be dated retrospectively. All other specific causes of dementia must be excluded through the clinical investigations in Table 5.2. Multi-infarct dementia presents with a history of stepwise deterioration as the patient experiences episodic strokes. In fact, this history is usually very difficult to document since there may be a very wide distribution of many small strokes. The resulting death of nerve cells may go undetected until very strategic areas of the brain are involved or until a major stroke occurs. There is often a history of hypertension.

The initial development and progression of the symptoms of dementia are extremely variable. Quite commonly, one particular cognitive deficit is found to dominate the clinical presentation although evidence for others may be found on closer examination. Examples of these clinical presentations are as follows: an amnestic syndrome with a relatively pure defect in memory; an aphasic syndrome with various language deficits; a parietal lobe syndrome with marked visual-spatial disorientation and apraxia; and, a frontal lobe syndrome dominated by personality changes and paranoid symptoms.

Memory Loss

Certain anatomical structures in the brain appear to be critical in the formation of new memories. These structures, closely related to the limbic system or "emotional brain", form a memory circuit of nerve cell fibres as follows: hippocampal gyrus of the temporal lobe, hippocampus, fornices, mammillary bodies, mammillo-thalamic tract, dorsomedial nucleus of the thalamus, and projections to various areas of the cortex where "memories" are stored. As previously noted, the disease process in Alzheimer's disease has a predilection for the hippocampal gyrus. The concentration of nerve cell loss in this critical area accounts for the memory loss as the cardinal feature of Alzheimer's disease.

The memory loss experienced by patients with Alzheimer's disease has been described as malignant as opposed to the more benign forgetfulness which occurs with normal senescence. The latter memory loss is characterized by the inability to recall relatively unimportant details of an experience (i.e. name of a person involved, the exact date, the location of the event) while the overall experience itself is not forgotten. In contrast, the malignant form of memory loss in Alzheimer's disease is characterized by impaired recollection of both the details and the entire events (i.e. the wedding of a child, the death of a spouse, a recent change in residence).

Figure 5.2 illustrates a simplified model for memory, defined as the mental processes of registration, retention, and retrieval (recognition and recall) of information. Appreciation of this model and the neuronal loss may facilitate understanding of the memory impairment experienced by the dementing patient. That understanding may in turn assist in the approach to clinical management by all clinical disciplines.

The first stage in memory involves the registration of the stimulus or information. For this to occur, the individual must be conscious and attending to the stimulus, those processes mediated by the reticular activating system in the brain stem. An impaired level of consciousness, anxiety, decreased

FIGURE 5.2

Memory: The Processes of Registration, Retention, and Retrieval (Recall and Recognition) of Information

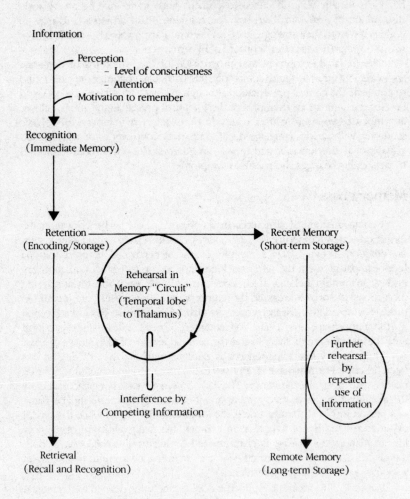

concentration and motivation, and many sedating drugs may all interfere with the process of registration, in turn leading to diminished retention of information. (It is in this way that the symptoms of depression may significantly impair memory processing leading to the appearance of pseudodementia.) Therefore, in management, anything that may improve the level of consciousness and attention to incoming stimuli may aid memory processing.

Registration of the stimulus is followed by the process of retention or encoding of the information which occurs in successive stages. The short-term stage of memory storage may be conceptualized as a physiological process. The information is transmitted by an electrochemical process along the nerve fibres in the memory circuit. A certain amount of incoming information is selected for retention. It is then rehearsed in this neuronal circuit, and is retained. An example of conscious rehearsal of new information occurs when looking up an unfamiliar telephone number and repeating it several times while picking up the phone and dialing the number. Rehearsal may be disrupted by the interference of new competing stimuli. Dementing patients appear to be particularly vulnerable to this interference because of an inability to focus attention on the material to be learned and remembered. It is this short-term stage of memory storage that is disrupted early in the course of Alzheimer's disease as the nerve cells in the memory circuit are destroyed. Thus, the patient is unable to remember new information or recent experiences. In order to cope with the progressive memory dysfunction, patients may develop techniques to permit the simplification, routinization, and repetition of information that must be used to perform daily activities. These become basic principles of management as well.

Of the many stimuli that pass through the short-term memory storage process, a few are selected for ongoing rehearsal and long-term storage. This is thought to become an anatomical process involving intra-neuronal protein synthesis for the storage of memories in the cortex. As Alzheimer's disease and other dementias progress to involve the loss of nerve cells in large areas of the cortex, long-term memories are lost.

The retrieval of information from memory storage involves the processes of recognition and free recall. Recognition is involved in selecting a response from a number of choices that are provided. Free recall is required when there is no cue to indicate the correct response.

Personality Change

The highest integrative functions of the cerebral cortex, those qualities considered uniquely human, are most vulnerable to disruption early in the course of dementia. The early loss of these functions is very subtle and may go undetected for many months until, in retrospect, someone close to the patient is able to notice a change. Four of these functions that constitute part of the structure of personality and which may become impaired in diseases of the cerebral cortex are as follows: (1) the capacity to express appropriate feelings and drives; (2) the capacity to employ mental mechanisms effectively for goals and achievements; (3) the capacity to maintain appropriate thresholds and tolerance for frustration and failure, and to recover appropriately from them; (4) the capacity to employ effective and modulated defense reactions.

The clinical manifestations of personality change in dementia are protean, ranging from accentuation of premorbid traits to behavior that is completely out of character. Some common examples of emotional and behavioral changes are:

1. Diminished interest in relationships, activities, goals, and achievements. Increasing self-concern.
2. Decreased concentration, task completion, and creativity.
3. Lability of affect—including anxiety, depression, irritability, outbursts of anger—in response to failure and environmental changes. They are worsened by a decreasing tolerance for frustration. With worsening, emotional responsiveness decreases with a flattening of affect and apathetic indifference.
4. Indecisiveness with the avoidance of new situations and initiation of activity involving choices.
5. Diminished social judgment with financial or sexual indiscretions.
6. Progressive neglect of personal grooming and hygiene, sometimes leading to urinary and fecal incontinence.
7. Restlessness and agitation or lethargy.
8. Increasing suspiciousness and distrust of others, including relatives and neighbors, sometimes leading to delusions of persecution or infidelity. The impaired memory contributes to this as misplaced or forgotten objects are believed stolen. A complete description of the paranoid symptoms which may develop during the course of dementia is presented in Chapter 7, Paranoid Disorders.
9. Impairments of specific cognitive functions such as speech and language, calculation, and visual-spatial orientation lead to related behavioral changes.
10. Increasing confusion in complex or unfamiliar circumstances.

Other Symptoms of Dementia

In addition to the above-noted symptoms and behavioral changes which are included in the DSM–III diagnostic criteria for dementia, patients may present with a number of other characteristic features of the syndrome.

Disorientation to time is very common early in the course of dementia and may progress from minor errors in the day of the week and month to gross errors in the year and season. Disorientation to place is also common with a similar range of errors. Disorientation to person may occur later in the course of deterioration and is evidenced by the inability to identify people, often close relatives.

The capacity to concentrate on a task involving a sequence of steps may be impaired. In addition, there may be considerable difficulty shifting attention from one stimulus to another so that the same thought or behavior pattern is repeated. This is referred to as perseveration. Alternatively, the patient may be unable to screen out irrelevant stimuli such that s/he is stimulus-bound or very distractible.

Insight as to the presence of declining cognitive ability is usually well-preserved early in the course of dementia but patients may not complain of cognitive impairment. Later in the course of illness, this insight is fortunately lost so the patient is not usually aware of profound disabilities once they develop.

(The examination for the symptoms of dementia is described in detail in Chapter 9.)

MANAGEMENT

If dementia is secondary to another disorder, the management involves the treatment of the underlying disease process. Unfortunately, there is no specific treatment that will interrupt the progressive deterioration caused by Alzheimer's disease. In addition, the dementia caused by some of the treatable diseases may not be completely reversible. Therefore, for most patients, management is palliative. To date, none of the etiological theories for Alzheimer's disease (i.e. acetylcholine deficiency, genetic, slow virus, autoimmune, aluminum concentration) have lead to specific effective treatments.

The general principle of management can be succinctly summarized as an attempt to increase the quality of life for the patient and to decrease the burden on the caregivers. It is useful to obtain as much information as possible about premorbid functioning and interests to acquire a general idea of the activity level and sociability of the patient prior to the onset of dementia. This provides some means to establish appropriate objectives in social management. For example, it is probably impossible to engage a passive, inactive, essentially asocial individual in new activities after the onset of dementia. On the other hand, if not depressed, the previously sociable and active individual can be assisted to maintain some of this lifestyle at least early in the course of illness.

The Patient

Concurrent medical, surgical, and psychiatric disorders should be treated vigorously. Unnecessary and/or potentially toxic medications should be discontinued since they may aggravate the cognitive dysfunction. Because patients are usually aware of their declining mental acuity well into the course of dementia, concurrent depression is very common. Therefore, adequate pharmacological or electroconvulsive therapy and supportive psychotherapy are essential. (A protocol for the use of antidepressants is presented in Chapter 11.) For patients with multi-infarct dementia, anti-platelet adhesiveness agents like acetylsalicylic acid may decrease the frequency of small vessel occlusion in the brain. Cerebral vasodilators (i.e. dihydroergotoxine mesylate) have not proven effective in altering the course of dementia.

Almost all patients at some time during their course of illness become irritable, agitated or frankly aggressive, with or without paranoid symptoms. In addition, sleep may be disrupted with the emergence of "sundowning" in which activity increases late at night. For all these conditions, the major tranquillizers or neuroleptics are preferable to the minor tranquillizers or sedative/hypnotic drugs which may have a disinhibiting effect on behavior. Very small dosages of neuroleptics are usually effective. (A protocol for the use of neuroleptics is also presented in Chapter 11.)

Patients whose aggression cannot be controlled pharmacologically or who wander from their residence must be restrained with the least restrictive but appropriate method. Dietary control and toilet training should be used to manage incontinence. The physical safety and financial competence of each patient should be assessed and appropriate management instituted. (These issues are addressed in further detail in Chapter 10 and Chapter 13.)

Information presented to the patient should be simplified and repeated frequently, such as repeated orientation, to reduce the ambiguity of situations. Sequences of information should be avoided because the patient may not be able to shift rapidly from concept to concept. Daily activities should be routinized and the amount of environmental change minimized. Relatively stable patients may deteriorate when their environment is changed such as on hospital admission or during a visit to a relative.

The Relatives and Other Caregivers

Dementia places an enormous psychological, social, and economic burden on families and other individuals involved in patient care. Even when outward appearances of normality are preserved early in the course, the witnessing of the cognitive decline is very distressing. Once established, the diagnosis should be explained and the various aspects of management should be discussed.

Relatives are quite often unable to appreciate the relationship between behavioral change and the underlying destruction of brain tissue. Therefore, some behavior is regarded as "psychological" in origin (and, hence, purposeful) and the patient is expected to exercise more self-control. In addition, patients are often expected to understand explicit verbal instructions or to comply with reasonable requests. Of course, this is impossible if the patient is aphasic or has lost insight as to the presence of the dementia. The failure of the patient to meet these expectations may lead to additional frustrations for the caregivers. Therefore, it is useful to provide a description of the underlying disease process to prevent the development of inappropriate expectations as the disease progresses.

Various community support services should be made available while the patient resides in a home with relatives. Such services should include supportive counselling. (Support services are described in Chapter 14 and Chapter 15.)

Residential placement must be considered when the mental state has deteriorated to the point where there is gross behavioral abnormality and the burden on the family becomes excessive. Patients are not to be maintained in the community at all costs, particularly in the presence of very aggressive/ assaultive behavior and/or regressed self-care such as frequent urinary and fecal incontinence. (See also Chapter 10.)

CONCLUSION

A considerable amount of neuronal loss and cortical atrophy may occur with little observable change in behavior since much of the cortex is "silent" with respect to activities of daily living. Indeed, there is no close correlation between the degree of cortical atrophy and the severity of dementia. However, this same loss of neurons may lead to "silent" abnormal behavior which may simply not come to the attention of others. Alternatively, small lesions in more critical areas may be manifested in much more visible behavior which readily comes to the attention of others. The progression of the neuronal loss in dementia is extremely variable and may be quite protracted, taxing the resources of both the patient and those who must provide care.

Also from Act Two, Scene Seven of *As You Like It*: "Thou seest we are not all alone unhappy: this wide and universal theatre presents more woeful pageants than the scene wherein we play in." It is hard to imagine a more woeful pageant than that of the progressive decline in cognitive function which is dementia. In the presence of this grim description of life's last scene, it is important to do whatever is feasible to improve the quality of life of the patient and to ease the burden of the family and other caregivers.

REFERENCES AND SUGGESTED READINGS

Adams R. D. and M. Victor. 1981. *Principles of Neurology*. 2nd ed. New York: McGraw-Hill.

American Psychiatric Association. 1980. *Diagnostic and Statistical Manual of Mental Disorders*. 3rd ed. American Psychiatric Association.

Arie T. 1973. "Dementia in the Elderly: Diagnosis and Management." *British Medical Journal*. 4: 540.

Chapman L. F. and H. G. Wolff. 1959. "The Cerebral Hemispheres and the Highest Integrative Functions of Man." *Archives of Neurology*. 1: 357.

Hachinski V. C., N. A. Lassen and J. Marshall. 1974. "Multi-infarct Dementia: A Cause of Mental Deterioration in the Elderly." *Lancet*. 2: 207.

Kral V. A. 1962. "Senescent Forgetfulness: Benign and Malignant." *Canadian Medical Association Journal*. 86: 257.

Martin B. A., E. G. Thompson and M. R. Eastwood. 1983a. "The Clinical Investigation of Dementia." *Canadian Journal of Psychiatry*. 28: 282.

Martin B. A., A. M. Peter and M. R. Eastwood. 1983b. "The Mental Status Examination for Dementia: A Review of Practice in a Psychiatric Hospital." *Canadian Journal of Psychiatry*. 28: 287.

Ropper A. H. 1979. "A Rational Approach to Dementia." *Canadian Medical Association Journal*. 121: 1175.

Thompson E. G. and M. R. Eastwood. 1981. "Survivorship and Senile Dementia." *Age and Ageing*. 10: 29.

Tomlinson B. E., G. Blessed and M. Roth. 1968. "Observations on the Brains of Non-demented Old People." *Journal of the Neurological Sciences*. 7: 331.

Tomlinson B. E., G. Blessed and M. Roth. 1970. "Observations on the Brains of Demented Old People." *Journal of the Neurological Sciences*. 11: 205.

Victor M. 1969. "The Amnesic Syndrome and Its Anatomical Basis." *Canadian Medical Association Journal*. 100: 1115.

Wells C. E. 1977. *Dementia*. 2nd ed. Philadelphia: R. A. Davis.

Wells C. E. 1978. "Chronic Brain Disease: An Overview." *American Journal of Psychiatry*. 135: 1.

Wells C. E. 1974. "Pseudodementia." *American Journal of Psychiatry*. 136: 895.

Yesavage J. A., J. R. Tinklenberg and L. E. Hollister et al. 1979. "Vasodilators in Senile Dementias." *Archives of General Psychiatry*. 36: 220.

6
Delirium

Donald A. Wasylenki, M.D., M.Sc., F.R.C.P. (C)

Delirium is a mental disorder characterized primarily by fluctuating clouding of consciousness. Since consciousness is necessary for cognitive processes to occur, there is a global cognitive dysfunction as well. Along with disordered attention, the patient manifests disorientation, impaired memory, poor judgment, lack of insight and intellectual impairment. Delirium is especially prevalent among patients with dementia, and nearly every physical illness can give rise to delirium in an elderly person.

Milder forms of delirium produce irritability and inattention. More severe forms lead to stupor and coma. Impaired consciousness is thus a contiuum, ranging from irritability and inattention through full-blown delirium to stupor and coma. Clouding of consciousness is described as a reduction in the clarity of awareness of the environment.

Table 6.1 lists the American Psychiatric Association diagnostic criteria for delirium.

Clouding of consciousness, disorientation and memory impairment, rapid onset, and fluctuating course are the hallmarks of delirium. Delirium must be differentiated from schizophrenia, schizophreniform and other psychotic disorders, and dementia.

It is estimated that between one-third and one-half of the hospitalized elderly are likely to be delirious at some point during admission. Roughly 25 percent of delirious elderly patients die within one month of admission. Fifty percent recover and are discharged, while approximately 25 percent become difficult to distinguish from the chronically demented. The occurrence of delirium must always raise the suspicion of an acute, reversible underlying pathology, and although some delirious states are self-limiting, others may be fatal if appropriate treatment is not instituted.

Detailed clinical examination usually enables a distinction to be made between delirium and dementia. However, demented patients may become

TABLE 6.1
Diagnostic Criteria for Delirium

A. Clouding of consciousness (reduced clarity of awareness of the environment), with reduced capacity to shift, focus, and sustain attention to environmental stimuli.

B. At least two of the following:
   (1) perceptual disturbance—misinterpretations, illusions, or hallucinations;
   (2) speech that is at times incoherent;
   (3) disturbance of sleep-wakefulness cycle, with insomnia or day-time drowsiness;
   (4) increased or decreased psychomotor activity.

C. Disorientation and memory impairment (if testable).

D. Clinical features that develop over a short period of time (usually hours to days) and tend to fluctuate over the course of a day.

E. Evidence, from the history, physical examination, or laboratory tests, of specific organic factor judged to be etiologically related to the disturbance.

American Psychiatric Association Diagnostic and Statistical Manual of Mental Disorders, Third Edition. Washington, DC, copyright APA 1980. Used with permission.

delirious and delirium may be a prelude to dementia. When a demented patient becomes physically ill, s/he may become delirious. In such cases the delirium must be recognized as separate from the dementia. This state of dementia with superimposed delirium has been called beclouded dementia, and is the most common cause of delirium on a general medical service. The term "sundowning", meaning the appearance of delirium at night, often applies to this state. Sundowning is thought to be due partly to the effects of fatigue, partly to the loss or blurring of familiar environmental cues, and partly to disordered wakefulness.

Characteristic clinical features distinguish delirium from dementia. In delirium, onset is acute, whereas in dementia it is often slow and insidious. Although both conditions may result in global cognitive impairment, the diagnosis of dementia is not made if the impairment is due to clouding of consciousness. The clouded, delirious patient often appears drowsy and is unable to focus attention. The severity of clouding and of intellectual impairment may fluctuate from hour to hour, or even during the course of a single examination. During lucid periods, cognition may be relatively intact. Such fluctuations in severity of impairment are not seen in dementia. Roth (1969) also points out that the mentation of the clouded patient may be more elaborate than in dementia. However, this will be less striking when delirium and dementia co-exist as cortical destruction with impoverishment has occurred, rather than simply disturbance of cortical function. As Roth notes,

> Psychic life in clouding is full, sometimes extravagantly so, but distorted: the patient lives in a private world of shifting experiences richly supplied with detail from the resources of a brain which

is essentially intact. He may imagine the ward to be, for instance,
a railway station or his place of work, and behave accordingly....
In dementia, by contrast, the patient lives in the actual world
but does so deficiently (1969, 712).

The phenomenon of double orientation, which is rare in dementia, also occurs
in delirium. The patient recognizes where s/he is; for example, in hospital,
but insists it is near some familiar place such as her/his home. Finally, severe
perceptual disturbance is much more common in delirium than dementia, with
vision affected to the greatest extent. Visual hallucinations and illusions occur
frequently.

   Table 6.2 outlines essential features which help to distinguish delirium
from dementia. However, none is pathognomonic of either condition.

TABLE 6.2
Differential Diagnosis of Delirium and Dementia

Feature	Delirium	Dementia
Onset	Rapid, often at night	Usually insidious
Duration	Hours to weeks	Months to years
Course	Fluctuates over 24 hours; worse at night; lucid intervals	Relatively stable
Awareness	Always impaired	Usually normal
Alertness	Reduced or increased; tends to fluctuate	Usually normal
Orientation	Always impaired, at least for time; tendency to mistake unfamiliar for familiar place or person	May be intact; little tendency to confabulate
Memory	Recent and immediate impaired; fund of knowledge intact if dementia is absent	Recent and remote impaired; some loss of common knowledge
Thinking	Slow or accelerated; may be dream-like	Poor in abstraction, impoverished
Perception	Often misperceptions, especially visual	Misperceptions often absent
Sleep-wake cycle	Always disrupted; often drowsiness during the day, insomnia at night	Fragmented sleep
Physical illness or drug toxicity	Usually present	Often absent, especially in primary degenerative dementia

Lipowski Z. J. 1983. "Transient Cognitive Disorders (delirium, acute confusional states) in
the Elderly." *American Journal of Psychiatry*. 140: 1426–1436.

CLINICAL FEATURES

Delirium has many causes. Thus, it is not strictly correct to speak of it as a clinical entity. Rather it is a complex of signs and symptoms which indicate that brain function is disrupted. The primary manifestations of delirium include:

1. Clouding of consciousness with global cognitive impairment
2. Restlessness and apprehension or apathy
3. Incoherent speech
4. Illusions, hallucinations, and delusions

The presence of these features in any patient calls for an immediate plan of action to control the acute situation, as well as energetic attempts to uncover the cause as quickly as possible.

Lipowski states that "Only the basic fact of global cognitive impairment is constant and diagnostic" in delirium (1967, 250). As noted previously, this global cognitive impairment is secondary to clouding of consciousness. Table 6.3 shows characteristics of clouding of consciousness. Impaired grasp of the environment is almost always present. The ability to comprehend relationships in the environment is lost. Attention is disrupted. There may be decreased attention span, fluctuations in attention, or difficulties in shifting attention from one area to another.

TABLE 6.3

Characteristics of Clouding of Consciousness

1. The person is awake.
2. Awareness is reduced.
3. Both immediate and recent memory are impaired.
4. Attention is disordered.
5. Thinking is more or less disorganized and thus altered.
6. Ability to match current information inputs against stored information resulting from past learning is diminished.
7. The person is unable to overcome this state by deliberate effort.

Lipowski Z. J. 1980. *Delirium: Acute Brain Failure in Man*. Springfield: Charles C. Thomas.

Disorientation and memory impairment are the key cognitive signs of delirium.

Disorientation may be for time, place, or person. It is tested by asking the patient a series of simple questions. Do you know what day it is? What date? What month? What year? Do you know where you are? The name of this place? What type of place this is? Where this place is located? Do you know who you are? Who I (examiner) am? What my job is? If delirium is severe, disorientation in all three spheres may occur. However the patient practically never loses the sense of personal identity.

Orientation for time is the first to be impaired and, as recovery progresses, the last to be restored. Temporal disorientation may be followed by impairment of orientation for place and for person. One of the characteristic manifestations of disorientation in delirium is a tendency to mistake unfamiliar places and persons for familiar ones. Thus, the disoriented patient may mistake the hospital room for the living room of his/her home or a hotel pub! Disorientation is a diagnostically useful but not absolute indicator of delirium. Disorientation as a sign may occur in many other clinical conditions. However, its occurrence in conjunction with clouding of consciousness is highly suggestive of delirium.

Impairment of memory occurs in nearly every delirious patient. In assessing memory in the elderly, it is important to distinguish between benign and malignant forms of amnesia. Benign amnesia is the inability to recall unimportant details associated with events, while the events themselves are remembered. Malignant amnesia is a rapidly progressive memory disorder characterized by the inability to recall recent events. Malignant amnesia, occurring in the absence of clouding of consciousness, is the hallmark of the dementias. However severe, recent memory loss also occurs in delirium as a result of clouding of consciousness.

Memory functions include registration, retention, and retrieval. Intact registration, or immediate memory, allows the holding of information for periods of seconds to a few minutes. An example is remembering a new telephone number for as long as it takes to dial. Registration requires an intact ability to attend. With clouding of consciousness and disordered attention, the registration function becomes impaired. Patients are unable to register a series of numbers long enough to repeat them back to an examiner. This is an important sign of clouded consciousness which helps to differentiate the delirious patient from the patient who is simply demented.

The retention function has short- and long-term components. Short-term retention is impaired in delirium. Its impairment results in memory loss for day-to-day events. In a test situation, patients with impaired short-term retention are unable to recall a name, address or color after three to five minutes, or to recall the names of five objects shown to them minutes before. They are, of course, unable to describe the events of the preceding day.

Retrieval, which is the ability to gain access to remote memories, may or may not be affected in delirium. The patient may be unable to report significant dates from his/her personal past history, or to recall the dates of important historical events. Retrieval is usually spared in mild to moderate cases of dementia, but may become impaired as the dementia progresses. (See also Chapter 9.)

Delirium, then, may involve impairment of all three memory functions, but the most characteristic impairment is in registration. In addition, there will be some degree of both anterograde and retrograde amnesia surrounding the delirious episode.

Restlessness and apprehension are common signs in delirium. In the early stages, sometimes described as incipient delirium, the patient becomes restless and ill at ease. S/he may become irritable and hypersensitive to light and noise. There may be an impression of bewilderment. This picture is usually transitory and may alternate with periods of apparent normality. As the delirium progresses, the patient may become increasingly fearful and/or aggressive. S/he may try to get out of bed and wander away. About 10 percent of the patients may display violence toward others. There is always the possibility that patients may hurt themselves or others while in this restless overactive state. In so-called occupational delirium, patients carry out complex motor movements associated with their work. In severe states of delirium, patients may make only fragments of purposive movements, and may spend time picking at clothing or rubbing blankets together. Tremors and choreiform movements may also occur. The sleep pattern is upset. The patient is most often drowsy by day and restless at night. Disordered wakefulness and sleep-wake cycle are among the essential features of delirium. Lipowski describes a typical elderly delirious patient as "... awake, restless, agitated, bewildered and often hallucinating during the night ..." (1983, 1437).

The emphasis on overactivity and restlessness as the rule in delirium may result from patient selection. Reduced activity is often observed in delirious patients. Some patients appear lethargic, drowsy, slowed down, and even immobilized. Because such patients are not disturbing, they often escape recognition. During the course of delirium, the same patient may show a gamut of motor behavior ranging from restlessness to extreme lethargy. Hyperkinetic and hypokinetic delirium have been described as variants. In contrast to the agitated restlessness of hyperkinetic delirium, a patient with the hypokinetic form will present with an apathetic, clouded state. Occasionally a patient may present with a mixture of the two forms.

Perceptual disturbances are also characteristic of delirium. These include illusions and hallucinations. Vision is usually affected to a greater extent than any other sensory modality. For example, a delirious patient may suffer the illusion that a coat hanging in a closet is a persecutory figure. The properties of surroundings are misperceived. A room may seem very large or very small, or the furniture may seem to move. Objects may be misidentified. A pattern on the wallpaper may appear to be writhing snakes or spots on the floor may appear to be crawling beetles. More complex illusions may be regarded as projections of personally meaningful symbols and fantasies onto environmental stimuli. Misinterpretations of stimuli in other sensory modalities are less usual but may occur. Sounds from a public address system, for example, may be misinterpreted as referring to the patient and incorporated into delusional thinking.

Hallucinations are perceptions which occur without relevant or adequate sensory stimulation. Delirious patients may see small animals or insects crawling about in the room in the absence of any wallpaper patterning or other stimuli. Hallucinations, like illusions, are usually visual and may be very simple, such as flashes, zigzags or spots of light, or complex such as fantastic kaleidoscopic visions involving people, animals, and other objects. The incidence of all types of hallucinations in cases meeting the criteria for delirium is in the range of 40 to 75 percent. Roughly two-thirds are visual and in about half of the patients, hallucinations occur only at night. It has been claimed that younger delirious patients hallucinate more frequently than older ones, and that certain types of delirium are more likely to cause hallucinations than others. Finally, it is common to observe hallucinations in one or two modalities occurring simultaneously and auditory hallucinations, alone or in combination with visual ones, occur in about 30 to 50 percent of cases.

Delusions also occur frequently in delirium, and may be closely connected with illusions and hallucinations. A delusion is a false belief not shared by others in the patient's environment and not in keeping with the patient's background. A paranoid attitude is common and the incidence of delusions in the delirious elderly is 40 to 55 percent. Lipowski states that "perhaps the most common delusion in delirium is belief in the reality of one's hallucinations" (1980, 125). Delusions in delirium tend to be transient and unstable, often being abandoned quickly and replaced by other delusions. Delusions of persecution are the most common type and many patients believe, at some point, that they are being persecuted. Delusions may also be grandiose, leading the patient to believe that s/he is some important person.

Incoherent speech occurs in delirium as a manifestation of interference with thought processes and content. The patient experiences difficulty in marshalling thoughts logically, coherently, and appropriately. Memories and associations become difficult to obtain, and inappropriate memories and associations appear in their place. The actual execution of speech may encounter the same difficulty. Patients become increasingly incoherent as delirium progresses. In mild delirium, speech may be characterized by vagueness, uncertainty and hesitancy, and the patient may acknowledge that s/he is having some difficulty thinking. At a later point, s/he begins to have significant difficulty in dealing with abstract concepts and conversation becomes limited and irrelevant. With progression, language becomes less coherent and comprehensible as the capacity to maintain attention increasingly diminishes. In the final stages of delirium, before stupor or coma intervenes, the patient's speech becomes entirely incoherent and muttering. S/he seems to be incapable of responding to even the simplest questions.

Several components of thinking are disturbed in delirium. Organization of thoughts is disrupted so that thinking is fragmented, illogical, and undirected. The flow of thoughts may be either retarded or accelerated. Concept formation is impaired so that thinking abstractly becomes difficult, and thought content may be impoverished or as noted above, delusional. All of these aspects of disturbed thinking contribute to the production of incoherence.

Signs of autonomic, especially sympathetic, nervous system arousal also occur in delirium. These are most marked in hyperkinetic delirium and represent the physiological concomitants of anxiety and fear. They include tachycardia, sweating, hypertension, dilated pupils, fever, flushing, and tremor. It should be noted however, that infections with fever may be a cause of delirium in the elderly and fever should not be dismissed simply as a result of increased arousal. Incontinence of urine and/or feces also occurs.

Secondary psychological disturbances also occur in delirium. These are disturbances of affect which arise in response to the primary cognitive impairment. The most common affective disturbances in delirium are anxiety, fear, and depression. Less often, euphoria, rage, or apathy may occur. These abnormal affects may be a function of the patient's personality structure, the nature of the organic illness causing the delirium, the effect on the limbic system, cultural factors, or the psychological stress of potentially life-threatening organic illness.

Classically the entire symptom picture in delirium follows a fluctuating course with lucid intervals. For short periods of time the patient will regain full awareness, only to lapse back into delirium. As noted, deterioration towards nightfall or nocturnal accentuation is a classical feature.

The electroencephalogram (EEG) may be extremely useful in the diagnosis and management of delirium. The earliest signs of delirium usually correspond with a slowing of brain wave activity of one to two cycles per second. With more severe disturbances, activity will usually slow from the normal 11 to 13 cycles per second to about 6 cycles per second. If the cause of the delirium is corrected, there is an increase in EEG activity corresponding to clinical improvement. In general, patients with delirium manifested by a decreased level of awareness show slowing of the EEG; in an agitated delirium, the EEG may be marked by low voltage, fast activity that is characteristic of intense arousal. In all cases, failure of the EEG to return to normal indicates that treatment is inadequate or incorrect.

Delirium tremens or DTs is a common and fairly typical example of delirium. It is seen frequently in elderly alcoholics. Ten percent of all chronic drinkers develop DTs, and the frequency with which the condition terminates in death makes it an important medical problem.

DTs usually start after a heavy drinker temporarily stops drinking. In the elderly, this may be due to hospitalization for physical illness. S/he becomes restless and fearful and develops an attitude of perplexity and bewilderment. This is followed by a progressive diminution of awareness. The condition progresses to a state of terror with disorientation. Initially sensory disturbances are visual illusions—s/he misinterprets what s/he sees. From illusions, s/he goes on to hallucinations—again, usually visual, and often of small objects or animals. By this time, s/he is in a dream world, losing contact with reality, and from there, if untreated, s/he may worsen to stupor and coma, and to death.

The patient with DTs looks disturbed. Restlessness and impulsivity, coupled with fear and poor judgment may result in suicide attempts. Speech is often incoherent. Clouding of consciousness and disorientation are obvious. The person tires easily and quickly becomes confused. The picture fluctuates and vacillates and the patient is emotionally labile. Invariably, the symptoms and signs worsen at night.

CAUSES

The underlying cause of delirium is interference with cerebral metabolism. This can come about in many ways. Brain metabolism depends on several factors including adequate blood supply from normal vessels carrying adequate amounts of glucose and oxygen. Anything which alters this balance can disturb brain function. In addition, cellular metabolism requires enzymes and co-enzymes derived from vitamins. Vitamin deficiency diseases may cause delirium. Furthermore, many metabolites such as ammonia, produced in hepatic failure, and acetone as well as other compounds produced in renal failure can interfere

TABLE 6.4

Common Causes of Delirium

Drugs
Alcohol
Infections
Cardiovascular Disorders
Cerebrovascular Disorders
Metabolic Disorders
Seizure Disorders
Head Injury
Post-operative States
Intensive Care Units
Pseudodelirium

with the normal functioning of brain tissue. Changes in electrolyte balance and many organic and inorganic compounds, including drugs and alcohol, can all affect cerebral metabolism. Delirium may also occur as a reaction to acute stress, relocation, sensory overload and deprivation, and sleep pathology. Lipowski suggests that when symptoms and signs of delirium occur in the absence of demonstrable organic causes, the term "pseudodelirium" be used (1983). He notes that 5 to 20 percent of elderly patients with apparent delirium will be found to be suffering from "pseudodelirium".

Ageing processes, addiction to alcohol or drugs, brain damage or disease, and impaired vision or hearing predispose the elderly to delirium. Almost any physical illness or adverse drug reaction may cause delirium in a predisposed elderly patient. Of 588 elderly patients admitted to six geriatric departments in England and Scotland, 68.2 percent were suffering from cognitive impairment with 24.5 percent being delirious. In an acute medical unit, 16 percent of 100 elderly patients admitted were delirious. A Canadian study of 71 patients over age 70 admitted to an acute medical unit found 32.8 percent to be mentally impaired of which 17.6 percent were delirious. Since brain function is under-evaluated, the true incidence is likely much higher (Fisher, 1982).

It must be kept in mind that in patients with any degree of dementia the amount of abnormality needed to produce delirium may be much less than would be considered normally necessary. For example, an elderly demented patient with the flu may go on to develop a mild pneumonia and become delirious. This is because decreased respiratory function has resulted in slightly less oxygen getting to the brain, disrupting an already compromised cerebral cortex. However, once the pneumonia clears and the brain is once again receiving adequate oxygen, the delirium disappears. In the majority of cases, delirium is a temporary, reversible condition.

Table 6.4 lists common causes of delirium. The most frequent causes of delirium are exogenous substances, principally drugs and alcohol. Both intoxication with and withdrawal from these substances may cause delirium. Alcohol intoxication is a very common cause of delirium. Estimates are that as many as 10 percent of those age 60 or older are heavy drinkers. Alcoholism and

TABLE 6.5
Drugs Which Commonly Cause Delirium

Anticholinergic drugs
  Antiparkinsonian drugs
  Tricyclic antidepressants

Tranquillizers and Hypnotics
  Major tranquillizers
  Minor tranquillizers
  Sleeping pills

Cardiac Drugs
  Digitalis
  Propanolol

Anticonvulsants

Antihistamines

Corticosteroids

Antibiotics

related physical illnesses often result in hospitalization. Thus, it is important in dealing with a delirious elderly patient to inquire about drinking habits, and to have a high index of suspicion with regard to alcoholism. Alcohol intoxication is characterized by maladaptive behavior due to recent ingestion of alcohol. This may include fighting, impaired judgment, or interference with social or occupational functioning. Physiological signs may include slurred speech, incoordination, unsteady gait, nystagmus, and flushed face. If the patient is delirious, attention will be impaired. States of pathological intoxication may also present with delirium. These states, described in *DSM-III* as alcohol idiosyncratic intoxication, are marked by extreme behavioral change—usually due to aggressiveness—after ingestion of a small amount of alcohol. There is usually subsequent amnesia for the period of intoxication.

Alcohol withdrawal states include delirium tremens, described above, and may include Wernicke's encephalopathy. Wernicke's encephalopathy is thought to be due to vitamin deficiency associated with prolonged, heavy use of alcohol. It is a neurological disease manifest by delirium, ataxia, eye-movement abnormalities, and other neurological signs. Gradually, with treatment, these manifestations subside, but a major impairment of memory, alcohol amnestic disorder, may remain.

Drug intoxications, withdrawal states, and adverse drug reactions commonly cause delirium in the elderly. Table 6.5 lists drugs which commonly cause delirium. Age-related changes in drug absorption, metabolism, and distribution as well as polypharmacy and high drug consumption in the elderly are all contributing factors. Many drugs and drug combinations, both licit and illicit, can be responsible for delirium. Anticholinergic drugs such as antiparkinsonian agents and tricyclic antidepressants are the most common drugs causing delirium in the elderly. Tranquillizers, both major and minor, and hypnotics (sleeping pills) should also be noted as common causes of delirium. Withdrawal from tranquillizing and hypnotic drugs also may cause delirium.

Acute intoxication with cardiac drugs such as digitalis and propanalol is a common cause of delirium because of the frequency with which these drugs are prescribed for elderly patients. Problems may arise in deciding whether an elderly delirious patient on digitalis is suffering from digitalis intoxication or from congestive heart failure, another common cause of delirium in the elderly. A physical examination should reveal the presence or absence of other signs of congestive failure. Other common medications which may cause delirium include anticonvulsants, antihistamines, levodopa, corticosteroids, cimetidine, and, in rare instances, antibiotics. Barbiturates can cause delirium from both intoxication and withdrawal. Fortunately, the use of barbiturates is increasingly rare, as the withdrawal state, in particular, is potentially lethal.

Among endogenous causes of delirium in the elderly, infections are the most common. As mentioned, fever secondary to infection may be the cause of delirium in the elderly. However, infections may also be afebrile, particularly in the early stages, but still cause delirium. It has been said that whereas fever is the most common sign of infection in the young patient, confusion is the most common sign in the elderly. Elderly patients with pre-existing dementia, which may or may not have been obvious before the onset of some infectious illness, are most susceptible to the development of acute delirious states. An apparently innocuous urinary tract infection may cause delirium in such a patient.

The most common infections causing delirium in the elderly are pneumonia and urinary tract infections. Infections such as pneumonia may be clinically silent until they are well-advanced and delirium may be the presenting feature. Lung diseases, mostly pneumonia, chronic bronchitis and emphysema, account for about 20 percent of cases of mental confusion in the elderly. Pneumonia is the most common post-operative complication in the elderly. Other infections which cause delirium less frequently include bacteremia, typhoid fever, viral infections, and intracranial infections such as encephalitis and meningitis. An unusual source of infection with delirium in the elderly that may easily be missed is subacute bacterial endocarditis, which usually originates from a sclerotic aortic valve.

Among medical conditions commonly causing delirium in the elderly, cardiovascular disorders are prominent. Delirium may follow a myocardial infarction, and delirium, following acute infarction, may represent an adverse prognostic sign. Cardiac arrhythmias may result in cerebral anoxia and delirium. Patients with chronic congestive heart failure may suffer episodes of delirium alternating with periods of restlessness. Such patients will be very vulnerable to delirium in response to any other factors which compromise cerebral functioning. As mentioned previously, it is important to rule out digitalis intoxication as the cause of delirium in elderly patients being treated for congestive heart failure. Although the widespread use of antihypertensive drugs has made hypertensive encephalopathy relatively uncommon, a rapid rise in blood pressure may cause delirium. In such cases, immediate attention must be paid to reducing blood pressure.

Cerebrovascular disorders also often present with delirium. Multi-infarct dementia, characterized by a stepwise deteriorating course with "patchy" distribution of deficits may present with episodes of delirium. Focal neurological signs and symptoms can usually be elicited. Delirium may also occur in transient ischemic attacks. These attacks are short episodes of cerebral dysfunction of vascular origin. There is no residual neurological deficit, although various signs of central nervous system dysfunction are notable throughout the episode. Usually the patient is amnestic for the period of the attack.

Many metabolic disorders may cause delirium, either alone or in combination with other factors. Metabolic disorders are among the most common causes of delirium in the elderly. The patient with delirium caused by a metabolic disorder may present with either an agitated or hypokinetic state.

As glucose is the main substrate of cerebral metabolism, hypoglycemia or hyperglycemia are potential causes of cerebral dysfunction and delirium. Hyperglycemia may be caused by poor treatment compliance in elderly diabetic patients or by other conditions such as infections, which tend to increase blood sugar levels in diabetes mellitus. Hypoglycemia may be caused by relatively rare organic syndromes such as islet-cell tumors of the pancreas or endocrine abnormalities, or it may be caused by exogenous agents such as alcohol, insulin and oral hypoglycemic drugs. According to Lipowski, symptoms of hypoglycemia may include "outbursts of anger, violence, paranoid delusions, catalepsy, dysarthria, ataxia, diplopia, vertigo, hemiparesis, and perceptual disturbances ..." (1980, 250). Delirium may last minutes to hours and is usually followed by amnesia.

Metabolic delirium may also occur as the result of organ failure. Hepatic or renal failure are common causes. The patient with hepatic failure may exhibit asterixis (flapping tremor of the outstretched hands) while renal insufficiency is characterized by myoclonus. In liver disease, metabolites are shunted past the liver and, therefore, may affect the brain. In renal failure certain metabolites cause delirium by blocking important biochemical pathways (Kreb's cycle).

In addition to hepatic and renal failure, hypoxia or hypercarbia due to severe lung disease may cause delirium. This is most common in patients with chronic obstructive pulmonary disease. Patients with chronic pulmonary insufficiency may gradually develop delirium. Delirium may also develop acutely in patients with chronic obstructive pulmonary disease as a result of acute exacerbations or respiratory failure. This may be due to infections or excessive sedation. Drowsiness is a common feature in delirium due to respiratory failure.

Other metabolic causes of delirium include disorders of sodium metabolism (hyponatremia or hypernatremia), disorders of calcium metabolism, (hypocalcemia or hypercalcemia), and metabolic or respiratory acidosis or alkalosis. These conditions, along with vitamin deficiency states which also may cause delirium, may arise as the result of poor fluid and/or food intake.

Delirium may occur following a seizure. Any delirious patient should be checked for evidence of a bitten tongue, cheek or lip, so that evidence of the occurrence of a seizure is not missed. Patients who become delirious after a seizure develop dazed reactions with deep confusion, bewilderment and anxiety or excitement, with hallucinations, fears, and possibly violent outbursts. Head injuries may also cause delirium and, especially in dealing with the elderly alcoholic, acute or subacute subdural hematoma should be considered. History and examination for evidence of a fall or other source of injury, with or without a period of lost consciousness, is essential. The classical clinical picture in subdural hematoma is rapidly fluctuating episodes of delirium and normal attention and alertness. Once a diagnosis is made, surgical intervention is required.

Post-operative delirium occurs frequently in elderly patients, although the actual incidence is unknown. The number of possible etiologic factors in post-operative delirium is extensive, but Lipowski (1980) lists the most common causes as cerebral hypoxia, electrolyte imbalance, drugs and alcohol and/or drug withdrawal syndromes. Heart surgery and eye surgery are especially likely to result in post-operative delirium. Postcardiotomy delirium frequently occurs 24 to 48 hours after surgery. There is a sudden onset of agitated behavior accompanied by disorientation and inability to grasp environmental events. The patient may become quite frightened and may interfere with monitoring equipment, try to get out of bed or even attempt to escape from the hospital. It is very important to rule out organic factors in such cases before attributing the disturbance to a psychological reaction.

Delirious states may develop among patients in medical intensive care units (ICUs). These states arise in response to severe physical illness, drugs and the alien environment of most ICUs with their lack of privacy, loss of normal human contact, disruption of the sleep-waking cycle, loss of awareness and day/night, physical discomfort, intimidating equipment, and the death of other patients. Severe anxiety characterizes patients' first response to intensive medical treatment. This anxiety is commonly dealt with by denial, by impulsive behavior, or by the intensification of chronic, defensive character traits. After about two days, the anxiety begins to yield to feelings of depression. The combination of anxiety-depression, the alien ICU environment, and the various medications the patient receives often leads to the development of delirium. The delirium is preceded by hyperalertness and irritability, and is usually relatively short-lived. It should be understood as comprising, to a great extent, a reaction to the experience of illness and to aspects of the experience of treatment.

As previously noted, Lipowski (1983) has recently introduced the term "pseudodelirium" to describe those states of apparent delirium in which no organic causative factor can be detected. He defines "pseudodelirium" as "a delirium-like transient cognitive disorder occurring in the absence of demonstrable organic causes" (Lipowski, 1983, 1435). He further states that the elderly, particularly those with some degree of dementia, are especially prone to exhibit pseudodelirium as a feature of an affective, schizophreniform, brief reactive, paranoid or atypical psychosis. It is well-known that stressful life events, such as bereavement, may cause apparent delirium in elderly patients, as may the experience of transfer and relocation. Although these phenomena are usually attributed to a non-specific decrease in stress-resistance mediated by the hypothalamus, they would seem to fall under the heading of pseudodelirium. Lipowski (1983) points out that in pseudodelirium, laboratory evidence of diffuse cerebral dysfunction is absent; the incidence is unknown; and clinical features have not been systematically studied. He concludes that this is an unexplored area of geropsychiatry and "one clamoring for research".

MANAGEMENT

Sir William Osler wrote of acute delirium, "... the indications for treatment are to procure sleep and to support the strength" (1892, 169). This rings as true today as it did in 1892.

Henry and Mann outline four tasks in the practical management of delirium:

1. Establish the presence of delirium on the basis of the clinical picture.
2. Recognize the situation as one which must be handled immediately until otherwise indicated.
3. Make all possible attempts to uncover the cause and course of the delirious state.
4. Carry out a combined program to (a) deal with the acute signs and symptoms and (b) remedy, wherever possible, the underlying condition (1965, 1160).

The mainstays of treatment of the acute situation are sedation, hydration and nutrition, nursing care, and environmental manipulation.

The management of delirious elderly patients should be as follows. Most importantly, the patient must be protected from harming him/herself or others and from physical exhaustion. Initial anxiety can sometimes be reduced by calm remarks and gestures from someone with whom the patient is familiar. Talking the patient down may produce some settling without having to resort to physical restraint or force.

If the patient is able to respond to interpersonal approaches and if the underlying cause of the delirium is understood and manageable, the situation may be handled in the patient's own home, without the added stress of relocation to a hospital. Familiar surroundings may have a very important calming effect which is lost when the environment is altered.

In talking down an elderly delirious patient, it is important to repeat identifying and orienting information. Simple, short, direct statements should be used. Conversation should relate to reference points for the patient such as occupation or special interests. The patient's emotional expression should be regulated by acknowledgment of how s/he feels followed by shifting of the focus to familiar, neutral topics. Tolerable amounts of information about what has happened should be provided, without emphasizing details that may be worrisome. Response to delusions should be neutral. The patient should be told that her/his beliefs are understood but not shared by others. Patients should not be encouraged to describe hallucinations in detail. It should be simply stated that the examiner cannot see small animals, etc., and that the patient is safe. If a patient becomes hostile, the examiner's perception of the situation should be calmly restated without argument. It is essential to maintain a calm, reassuring, optimistic manner, even with the most agitated, hyperactive, delirious patient.

If the patient cannot be settled using interpersonal approaches, it may be necessary to achieve sedation with tranquillizing medications. Whenever possible, a psychiatric consultation should be obtained. Psychiatrists working on medical and surgical wards have more familiarity with delirium and its management than other physicians. Together with other organic mental disorders, delirium accounts for about 20 percent of general hospital psychiatric consultations.

To achieve sedation, major tranquillizers, also known as antipsychotic drugs, are the drugs of choice. Minor tranquillizers may also be used but are usually less effective. Drug dosage should be based on factors such as the patient's size and history of drug responsiveness and the suspected underlying cause of the delirium. If antipsychotic drugs are used properly, they help to control the clinical picture without causing undesirable drowsiness by decreasing agitation and eliminating hallucinations and other psychotic symptoms. A small dose should be given initially to test the patient's responsiveness. Then the dose should be increased until the desired control is obtained without excessive drowsiness or other side effects. The patient must be responsive and co-operative during the day and able to sleep, or at least rest comfortably, at night. Therefore tranquillizing medication should be given in the early evening and repeated in several hours if necessary. This regimen will often eliminate sundowning if it has occurred. Often the use of 10 to 25 mg of thioridazine in the early evening is sufficient to control an elderly delirious patient over a 24-hour period. For patients who are combative or assaultive, haloperidol, 1 to 5 mg, has been recommended. Medication may be tapered and discontinued after several days of normal cognitive functioning. (See also Chapter 11.)

Hydration and nutrition must also be addressed in the management of the acute state. If the patient has shown evidence of dehydration or electrolyte imbalance, this should be corrected with appropriate intravenous infusions. Massive doses of B vitamins, especially thiamine, are very important in withdrawal syndromes. Dietary supplements should be made available as soon as the patient is able to begin eating.

While the underlying cause of delirium is being investigated, supportive nursing and environmental measures must be taken to deal with disturbed behavior and restlessness. If the patient is acutely disturbed, s/he should be kept on constant observation. With some degree of settling, frequent checks with reassurance should suffice. The patient should be in a room near nursing personnel. If possible, a relative should stay with the patient. If the patient requires eyeglasses or a hearing aid or an interpreter, they should be provided. The patient should be positioned so as to maximize her/his ability to receive sensations. A calendar, a clock, and familiar objects should be placed in easy view and a light should be left on at night. A simple chart of the day's activities may help some patients. Face-to-face contact is important in communicating with delirious patients, and the patient should be addressed consistently, using the most familiar and appropriate name. In addition to a light at night, nocturnal accentuation can be reduced by leaving a radio on quietly and providing more contact for the patient.

Patients who are extremely delirious and agitated may be safest with their mattress on the floor at night to prevent injury from attempts to get out of bed. For mildly confused patients, side-rails may suffice. Mittens and restraints may be necessary to protect severely agitated patients, but should seldom be necessary in the absence of severe agitation. An alternative to restraining patients in bed is to place them in a deep chair that is difficult to get out of and to put a table in front as a form of restraint. During the day the patient can be walked and can sit in a geriatric chair with a tray, lap tying if necessary. However, wherever possible, restraint should be avoided. Restraining a disoriented, fearful, physically ill elderly patient often exacerbates rather than helps to settle the agitated state, and struggles against restraints may lead to rapid exhaustion with increased levels of delirium.

Elderly patients may require a long time to recover normal mental functioning after an episode of delirium. Techniques to enchance return of the patient's control over self and the environment should be employed. These include informing and reminding her/him of where s/he is, how s/he got there, what has happened to her/him and what is expected of her/him. Decision-making should be returned gradually, beginning with simple things such as the menu, activities, bathing, sleeping, and progressing to decisions about treatment. All staff must be prepared to provide accurate information, and the patient should be informed of the diagnosis and prognosis, especially if full recovery is expected. Full recovery should not be ruled out too quickly, as often it requires an extended period of convalescence. Finally, ongoing careful attention to medications, physical health, and social and psychological circumstances in the elderly patient should allow for the prevention of full-blown delirious conditions presenting as medical emergencies.

The systematic investigation of the cause of a delirious patient's condition is properly addressed in textbooks of internal medicine and will not be dealt with in detail here. Suffice it to say that delirium in an elderly patient must always raise the suspicion of an underlying organic pathology. A thorough history and physical examination is necessary, including careful assessment of the patient's level of consciousness. As clinical signs are sometimes unclear, and as two or more causes of delirium may co-exist, a widespread biochemical investigation is indicated in most cases. It should include the following:

—   blood and urine cultures
—   WBC and differential count
—   ESR
—   serum creatinine
—   BUN and electrolytes
—   serum calcium and magnesium
—   liver function tests
—   blood gases
—   urine and blood screening for drugs and alcohol
—   chest and skull x-rays

An EEG, brain scan, and examination of the CSF may also be necessary. Provided the underlying condition is amenable to treatment and can be brought under some measure of control, most delirious states should be considerably improved within 48 hours.

REFERENCES AND SUGGESTED READINGS

American Psychiatric Association. 1980. *Diagnostic and Statistical Manual of Mental Disorders*. 3rd ed.

Bayer N. 1983. "Delirium." *Medicine North America*. 33: 3100.

Bayne J. R. 1978. "Management of Confusion in Elderly Persons." *Canadian Medical Association Journal*. 118: 139.

Dunn T. and T. Arie. 1973. "Mental Disturbance in the Ill Old Person." *British Medical Journal*. 2: 413.

Engel G. L. and J. Romano. 1959. "Delirium, a syndrome of Cerebral Insufficiency." *Journal of Chronic Diseases*. 9: 260.

Fisher R. H. 1982. "Acute Confusional States in the Elderly." *Modern Medicine of Canada*. 37: 192.

Gaitz C. M. and P. E. Baer. 1971. "Characteristics of Elderly Patients with Alcoholism." *Archives of General Psychiatry*. 24: 377.

Henry W. D. and A. M. Mann. 1965. "Diagnoses and Treatment of Delirium." *Canadian Medical Association Journal*. 93: 1156.

Kimball C. P. 1977. "Psychosomatic Theories and Their Contributions to Chronic Illness." *Psychiatric Medicine*. Ed. G. Usdin. New York: Brunner/Mazel Inc.

Kral V. A. 1962. "Senescent Forgetfulness: Benign and Malignant." *Canadian Medical Association Journal*. 86: 257.

Lipowski Z. J. 1967. "Delirium, Clouding of Consciousness and Confusion." *Journal of Nervous and Mental Diseases*. 145: 227.

Lipowski Z. J. 1980. *Delirium: Acute Brain Failure in Man*. Springfield: Charles C. Thomas.

Lipowski Z. J. 1983. "Transient Cognitive Disorders (delirium, acute confusional states) in the Elderly." *American Journal of Psychiatry*. 140: 1426.

Osler W. 1892. *Principles and Practice of Medicine*. New York: D. Appleton and Co.

Ropper A. H. 1979. "A Rational Approach to Dementia." *Canadian Medical Association Journal*. 121: 1175.

Roth M. R. and D. H. Myers. 1969. "The Diagnosis of Dementia." *British Journal of Hospital Medicine*. 114: 705.

Simon A. and R. B. Cahan. 1963. "The Acute Brain Syndrome in Geriatric Patients." *Psychiatric Research Report*. 16: 8.

Steinhart M. J. 1979. "Treatment of Delirium—A Reappraisal." *International Journal of Psychiatry in Medicine*. 9: 191.

Taylor G. and K. Doody. 1979. "Psychosomatic Issues: Psychiatric Consultations in a Canadian General Hospital." *Canadian Journal of Psychiatry*. 24: 717.

Wolff H. G. and D. Curran. 1935. "Nature of Delirium and Allied States." *Archives of Neurology and Psychiatry*. 33: 1175.

7

Paranoid Disorders

Donald A. Wasylenki, M.D., M.Sc., F.R.C.P. (C)

The essential features of paranoid disorders are persistent persecutory delusions. A delusion is a false belief maintained in spite of evidence to the contrary, and not ordinarily accepted by members of the patient's family, culture, or social group. Persecutory delusions in paranoid disorders may be simple or elaborate, and usually involve a single theme or series of connected themes. Examples of persecutory delusions include beliefs that one is being conspired against, cheated, spied upon, maligned, poisoned, or drugged. In delusional jealousy, the patient believes that his/her mate is unfaithful, and evidence is collected to justify the delusion.

Delusions are often preceded or accompanied by ideas of reference. These are false beliefs that the activities of others have personal reference, usually of a derogatory character, to the patient. Patients may believe that the lyrics of songs on radio or television broadcasts or newspaper reports refer directly and personally to them.

Paranoid disorders are often associated with feelings of resentment and anger which may lead to violence. Paranoid individuals rarely seek treatment, but are usually brought by friends, relatives, officials, or the police. Age of onset tends to be middle or late adult life, and the natural course of most paranoid disorders is chronic with few remissions or exacerbations. Intellectual and occupational functioning may be maintained, but social and marital functioning are often severely impaired. Paranoid disorders are thought to be relatively rare, although a large Scandinavian study found paranoid psychoses in 12 percent of admitted patients over a three-year period (1958 to 1961). Among the elderly, 10 percent of admissions fall into this category. Paranoid symptoms occur frequently in dementia. In nearly all paranoid psychoses in old age, females predominate markedly. Men account for 5 to 25 percent of patients with this diagnosis.

THE CONTINUUM OF PARANOID CONDITIONS

According to the American Psychiatric Association's Diagnostic and Statistical Manual, paranoid disorders include paranoia, shared paranoid disorder, acute paranoid disorder and atypical paranoid disorder.

In paranoia, the essential feature is the insidious development of a permanent and unshakable delusional system with preservation of clear and orderly thinking. In shared paranoid disorder, the essential feature is a persecutory delusional system that results from a close relationship with another person who already has a disorder with persecutory delusions. The delusions are at least partly shared. In acute paranoid disorder the essential features are persecutory delusions of relatively sudden onset, commonly seen in individuals who have experienced drastic changes in their environment such as immigrants and refugees. Atypical paranoid disorder consists of persecutory delusional states not classified in other categories. Many paranoid states in the elderly are classified as atypical paranoid disorder mainly because the delusions are often accompanied by hallucinations.

In addition to the above conditions, paranoid disorders include, at the ends of a continuum of severity, paranoid personality disorder and paranoid schizophrenia.

Individuals with paranoid personality disorder may show paranoid ideation or pathological jealousy, but there are no delusions. Such individuals may have a greater likelihood of developing persecutory delusions later in life.

These people are hypersensitive, suspicious, rigid, and self-important. They tend to blame others for their misfortunes and to ascribe evil motives to people. They are jealous and envious and have great difficulty in maintaining relationships. However, these personality traits are stable over time, and disabling pathology in the form of full-blown paranoid disorders with persecutory delusions and hallucinations may only develop late in life, if at all.

Cognitive styles characteristic of paranoid individuals have been described. Some are cognitively constricted and apprehensively suspicious. Others are grandiose and aggressively suspicious. The paranoid cognitive style is characterized by suspicious thinking, loss of reality sense, and an intense need for autonomy. Suspicious thinking focusses on the search for clues. Attention is rigidly directed to the discovery of the real meaning of things. This real meaning is some confirmation of an intense, biased belief system. The paranoid individual has actively scanning and searching attention. S/he is hypersensitive and hyperalert and only sees what s/he is looking for. Loss of reality occurs because s/he misses the plain face value of things. In a casual conversation, for example, s/he is listening for signs of what the other person really thinks, and has little interest in the actual content of what is said. S/he thus loses a sense of proportion. S/he may agree that something has happened, but not on the meaning of what has happened. Projection, the ego defence mechanism which results in attribution to external figures of feelings and thoughts that are intolerable to oneself, may crystallize the biased expectancy into some concrete shape. This type of cognition is immune to correction as the paranoid person "sees so much that is not there" (Shapiro 1965, 541).

The drive for autonomy is a defensive vigilance, keeping the person in readiness for an anticipated emergency. The paranoid individual creates and maintains a kind of internal police state. S/he watches, curbs, controls, and steers her/his behavior. Whatever s/he does has a purpose and s/he assumes this of other people as well. S/he is always fearful of being subjugated by some external force. Danger lies in giving in passively to some authority. Thus, paranoid individuals are extremely guarded people who experience life as a constant round of battles.

At the other end of the continuum of severity of paranoid conditions lies paranoid schizophrenia. These patients suffer from bizarre persecutory or grandiose delusions and hallucinations. Typically these hallucinations are auditory and consist of two or more voices discussing the patient in the third person. In addition, patients with paranoid schizophrenia manifest schizophrenic thought disorder which often results in incoherence. Delusions of control and thought broadcasting, withdrawal, and insertion occur. The experience of being controlled by alien forces suggests schizophrenia rather than paranoid disorders. Also, delusions in schizophrenia are more likely to be fragmented and malleable rather than systematized as in paranoid disorders. Elderly paranoid schizophrenic patients often become "bag people" wandering the streets with all of their belongings. With age, symptom intensity diminishes and when acute exacerbations do occur, less medication is needed to restore equilibrium and lower doses are often adequate for effective maintenance. It has been noted that with increasing age and chronicity in schizophrenic samples, paranoid symptomatology tends to disappear. Many patients who develop paranoid schizophrenia in middle age shift from paranoid to nonparanoid status with increasing chronicity.

Psychological mechanisms underlying paranoid states are denial and projection. Denial is a primitive defence mechanism by which some powerful experience or impulse is kept out of conscious awareness. Projection is the process of attributing to another person feelings, thoughts, or wishes that belong to oneself. Thus, an elderly person with some degree of memory impairment may deny any difficulties in remembering things. When something cannot be located, s/he will attribute the loss to someone else, perhaps accusing a janitor of stealing. In many cases, particularly among elderly individuals, what are denied are feelings of worthlessness. If the denial is maintained and projection is utilized then paranoid states develop (i.e. It is not my fault, therefore it must be his/her fault). If denial is not maintained, depression may occur. In the elderly, one often sees paranoid reactions to losses of objects or functions which decrease self-esteem. It has been suggested that as the entire ageing process is a sustained onslaught on self-esteem, states of paranoia are more easily provoked.

CLINICAL FEATURES

Roth (1955) described a group of patients whose first illness occurred late in life and in whom paranoid delusions and hallucinations were the most prominent features. He called this condition "late paraphrenia" to emphasize what he felt to be a close association of the illness to schizophrenia, while at the same time noting its distinctive features (Roth 1955). Late paraphrenia is mainly confined to women and accounts for 8 to 9 percent of female first admissions to psychiatric hospitals over the age of 65.

Late paraphrenia differs from classical schizophrenia in that deterioration of the personality does not occur. In addition, genetic factors are not nearly as prominent as in the etiology of schizophrenia. However, schizoid and paranoid personality traits occur frequently in the premorbid personality and there is an excess of unmarried individuals and married individuals with low fertility among late paraphrenic patients. These features are also associated with schizophrenia. There are other etiological factors which are not associated with schizophrenia. About one-third of late paraphrenics are deaf, a proportion are blind, and in some cases, severely stressful circumstances are associated with the onset of symptoms.

Late paraphrenic patients are often found living in extreme isolation from others. This may not be wholly self-induced as they have been found to have fewer surviving siblings, smaller families, fewer surviving children, and a higher incidence of deafness and other sensory defects. As noted, stressful life events often contribute to the onset of the illness.

Paranoid or schizoid premorbid personality traits or disorders are characteristic of many late paraphrenics and are probably an important cause of increasing social isolation with advancing age. Those who are parents are often described by their children as cold and unloving. Marriages often take place late in life, are unusual in character, and are marked by sexual difficulties and jealousy.

In the majority of cases of late paraphrenia, two stages may be defined in the development of the illness. The first takes the form of accentuation of previous paranoid or schizoid personality traits. The patient may become irritable and suspicious, seclude himself/herself, refuse callers, and develop ideas of reference. The police or other officials may be contacted with complaints about relatives or neighbors. The next stage begins with the onset of auditory hallucinations. Threatening voices, screams, shouts, or obscene words may be heard. Relatives or hostile neighbors may be held responsible. At this point, medical-psychiatric intervention is often obtained.

Hallucinations are often more disturbing at night without evidence of clouding of consciousness. Figures or faces may appear. Intruders may be detected on the roof or in the hallways. Delusions may arise abruptly. For example, a patient may accuse a man she hardly knows of molesting her at night. Life may be made intolerable by threats heard through the walls. A patient may go so far as to barricade himself/herself in a room or in a house and, if undiscovered for some time, become a recluse.

In place of the usual systematized persecutory delusions, there may be erotic, hypochondriacal, or grandiose delusions. Affective changes characteristic of schizophrenia are seldom seen and incoherent speech is exceptional, occurring only in cases of long duration. Patients are lucid with clear consciousness and cognitive defects are uncommon.

As noted, the illness pursues a chronic course and deterioration is uncommon. The overall expectation of life in late paraphrenic patients is very close to that of the general population of comparable age. The majority of patients respond to antipsychotic medication but continue to have difficulties in interpersonal relationships and remain isolated. Late paraphrenia must be distinguished from affective disorder with paranoid features and from paranoid states in patients suffering from delirium and/or dementia. In delusional depression, the delusional patient feels a great deal of self-reproach and the behavior of imagined persecutors is accepted as justified. These features are not present in late paraphrenia. In addition, six premorbid characteristics differentiate elderly paraphrenic patients from those with affective psychoses. These are presented in Table 7.1.

TABLE 7.1

Premorbid characteristics differentiating elderly paraphrenic patients from those with affective psychoses

1. Paraphrenic patients more likely to have a schizoid premorbid personality
2. Paraphrenic patients more likely to be childless or to have only one surviving child
3. Precipitating events more likely in the onset of illness for affective patients
4. Social deafness more likely in paraphrenic patients
5. Family history of mental illness twice as common in affective patients
6. Paraphrenic patients more likely to be in social classes IV and V.

Adapted from Kay D. W. K., A. F. Cooper and R. F. Garside et al. 1976. "The Differentiation of Paranoid from Affective Psychoses by Patients' Premorbid Characteristics." *British Journal of Psychiatry.* 129: 207.

With regard to differentiation from paranoid states associated with organic disorders, in late paraphrenia the deterioration of cognitive functions and personality seen in dementia does not occur and delusions and hallucinations develop in a setting of clear consciousness, as opposed to the clouding characteristic of delirium.

Following Roth's (1955) early work, Post (1966) observed elderly patients with late onset of delusions and hallucinations. He recognized three paranoid conditions in elderly patients: paranoid hallucinosis, schizophreniform illness and schizophrenia. He regarded these as "three grades of strength with which schizophrenic ways of experiencing and thinking emerge only late in life ..." (Post 1966, 121).

Paranoid hallucinosis or simple paranoid psychosis tends to be the least disruptive form of paranoid disorder in the elderly, and may remain entirely unnoticed. In many cases it is associated with deafness. Often the patient feels molested by talk. The patient usually suffers from one or two commonplace delusional beliefs, often associated with family members or neighbors. Personality functioning is not seriously disrupted. Such patients are often identified through complaints to the police, disputes with neighbors or the development of reclusiveness. The symptoms of this condition may disappear temporarily if the patient is removed from his/her usual isolated environment to live with family, friends, or in hospital.

In schizophreniform illnesses, the clinical picture is characterized by a more general disturbance of mental functioning. In addition to delusions and auditory hallucinations, the patient develops more florid and bizarre symptoms. These may include beliefs that gas and electricity supplies are being interfered with or that the patient is being subjected to special rays. The patient often becomes very distressed as the symptoms become more elaborate, and may call for help. The imagined persecutors become more powerful and more frightening than in paranoid hallucinosis. For example, rather than scheming or envious relatives or friends, gangs of thieves, the mafia, or communist agents threaten the patient.

In schizophrenic states the paranoid illness of late life displays classical signs and symptoms of paranoid schizophrenia. Schneiderian first-rank symptoms of schizophrenia are often prominent. The most common and most striking of these are auditory hallucinations discussing the patient in the third person. The patient reports hearing conversations referring to him/her by name or more often by the term "he" or "she". Other first rank symptoms include feelings of influence and passivity, thought control, thought insertion, and thought broadcasting. Whereas patients with paranoid hallucinosis or schizophreniform illnesses tend to calm down considerably when removed from their home surroundings, patients exhibiting a schizophrenic picture will fail to experience any remission on removal to a hospital or other sheltered situation. Among 93 patients over the age of 60 with persistent persecutory states first arising after the age of 50, there were 21 with paranoid hallucinosis, 37 with schizophreniform illnesses and 34 with symptoms of paranoid schizophrenia. On a three-year follow-up, the symptomatology of individual patients remained consistent and was not progressive.

Although Post (1973) divides the late life paranoid states into three syndromes, his observations are essentially in agreement with Roth's (1955) early description of late paraphrenia. No clear differences with regard to etiology or response to antipsychotic medication emerged among the three groups. The essential features of these conditions are summarized in Table 7.2.

Scandinavian investigators have tended to emphasize the reactive element in late life paranoid disorders and to differentiate these disorders from schizophrenia. Ageing itself is seen as predisposing to the development of paranoia as it results in such things as membership in a disadvantaged group, loneliness, isolation, detachment, faulty perception, and misinterpretation. Paranoia in the elderly is seen as by no means pathognomonic of schizophrenia. A psychologically traumatizing event is often causative, and when the conflict lessens, so does the psychosis. In a Scandinavian follow-up study comparing paranoid patients with paranoid schizophrenic patients, outcome was far better for the paranoid patients. Almost 90 percent of the schizophrenic group became chronically ill versus less than 25 percent of the paranoid group. Good prognostic factors for these patients were "being married, female, having a family history of psychoses, hypersensitive premorbid personality, older at onset, acute onset

TABLE 7.2

Essential features of late life paranoid states

1. First episode of illness occurs late in life.
2. Delusions and auditory hallucinations are the most prominent features.
3. Women are much more commonly affected.
4. There is little deterioration of the personality.
5. Premorbid personality is schizoid or paranoid.
6. Genetic factors are less prominent than for early onset schizophrenia.
7. Patients are unmarried or married with low fertility. There are few surviving siblings. Marriages are characterized by sexual difficulties and jealousy.
8. Sensory defects (deafness and blindness) and social isolation are common.
9. Illness pursues a chronic course with little deterioration.
10. Symptoms respond to antipsychotic medication.

Adapted from Roth M. R. and F. Post.

and depressive content or ideas of reference." Poor prognostic factors were "schizoid premorbid personality, insidious onset, no precipitating factors, hallucinations, ideas of influence, depersonalization and derealization" (Rettersol 1970, 265).

A recent study of late onset psychoses attempted to test the usefulness of *DSM-III* diagnostic criteria for elderly patients with hallucinations or delusions. Patients had their first manifestation of mental disorder after age 65 and no history of any major mental illness before age 65. The prevalence of late onset psychosis among 880 patients admitted to a geropsychiatry unit was 8 percent (N=70). Twenty-five patients had major affective disorder, 30 had organic mental disorder, and 15 had a primary psychotic disorder. Only 9 of the 15 met *DSM-III* criteria for paranoid disorders or atypical paranoid disorder. The prevalence figure of 1.7 percent for primary psychotic disorder is considerably lower than earlier estimates in the range of 4 to 8 percent and the study also highlights the diagnostic difficulty posed by attempting to apply *DSM-III* criteria to elderly paranoid patients. Five of nine patients were excluded from the category of paranoid disorders because of the presence of auditory hallucinations, a prominent feature of late paraphrenia as described by Roth (1955) and Post (1966). No other features differentiated the patients with hallucinations from those without.

DIFFERENTIAL DIAGNOSIS

Paranoid features such as ideas of reference, delusions, and hallucinations occur in clinical conditions other than late paraphrenia or the three types described by Post (1973). The most common conditions include dementia, delirium, and depression. In these conditions, paranoid features are secondary to the underlying disorder, but these features respond to treatment with antipsychotic medication regardless of the primary condition.

Paranoid Symptoms in Dementia

Dementia is characterized by progressive intellectual impairment. The hallmark is recent memory defect. A paranoid-hallucinatory syndrome may develop in the very early stages of dementing illnesses such as Alzheimer's disease, before clear signs of organic impairment become detectable. This is associated with subjective feelings that the world is becoming overwhelming. These feelings are thought to arise in response to the initial internal realization, conscious or unconscious, of declining cognitive abilities. As intellectual impairment increases in dementia, the syndrome of paranoid forgetfulness may develop. Typically this involves a suspicious, aloof, socially isolated, elderly individual who in old age, with increasing memory impairment and disorganization, begins to hide important objects and then cannot find them again. The development of delusions of theft, often involving innocent people with whom s/he is in regular contact then occurs. Most commonly there are no hallucinations in this condition. The paranoid symptoms do not respond to medications but they may respond to simple, frequent reassurance and reminding, as well as to environmental manipulations.

More often the patient's intellectual abilities, self-care, orientation, and memory are noticeably impaired for some time before paranoid features develop. False accusations and verbal or physical attacks may occur and paranoid ideation may be quite marked. Habitually jealous individuals who develop dementia may develop delusions of marital infidelity and will actually assault their spouse. Paranoid features in demented patients are often accentuated towards the end of the day and may include both delusions and hallucinations. Delirium must be ruled out by assessing the individual's level of consciousness. Even when there is a clear underlying dementia, any paranoid overlay usually responds to relatively small doses of antipsychotic medication. If the paranoid features do occur at a regular, predictable time of day, then medication should be given one to two hours before the symptoms have been observed to occur.

Structured and persistent paranoid symptoms occur only during the less advanced stages of dementia and probably most frequently in persons with previous abnormal personalities. At a latter stage, severe dementia is incompatible with all but very fragmented paranoid beliefs or experiences. As dementia progresses, delusions become vague, loosely connected, unsystematized, and often arise from poverty of grasp. There is gross deterioration of personality and intellect. In multi-infarct dementia, paranoid ideas sometimes occur and may be more systematized than in Alzheimer's disease, but the condition shows marked fluctuations. There may also be focal neurological signs. As a final point, the prevalence of dementia among patients who present with paranoid symptoms is no higher than in mentally healthy old people. Paranoid symptoms with onset in late life should not be interpreted as signalling the onset of dementia in the absence of signs of intellectual impairment. On the other hand, as noted, paranoid symptoms quite often do complicate progressive dementing conditions.

Paranoid Symptoms in Delirium

The essential feature of delirium is a clouded state of consciousness, usually manifest by difficulty in sustaining attention, sensory misinterpretation, and a disordered stream of thought. Perceptual disturbances are common and result in various misinterpretations, illusions, and hallucinations. There is often both a delusional conviction of the reality of hallucinations and an emotional and behavioral response in keeping with their content. Delirious patients often become disoriented, and this in combination with visual and other types of hallucinations may lead to the development of persecutory ideas which are always fleeting and fluctuating, and which are not exaggerated into any system of paranoid beliefs. Paranoid experiences however, may become very frightening to the delirious patient leading to aggressive or agitated panic behaviors. It is most important to be aware that delusions and hallucinations in delirious states occur in a setting of clouding of consciousness and not, as in other disorders, in clear consciousness. Paranoid and other symptoms of delirium clear rapidly when the underlying etiologic condition is remedied. If however, behavioral control is necessary before remedial measures can be effected, then small amounts of antipsychotic medication are usually effective. (Other aspects of the management of delirium are discussed in Chapter 3.)

Organic delusional syndrome is a condition between delirium and dementia. The essential feature is the presence of delusions that occur in a normal state of consciousness and that are due to a specific organic factor. Mild cognitive impairment is often observed and impairment of social and occupational functioning is usually severe. When the physical disorder producing this syndrome is not reversed, these states begin to shade into those associated with dementia. In the elderly, the most important causes of this syndrome are excessive or prolonged doses of numerous drugs and prolonged hypoxia due to cardiopulmonary disease.

Paranoid Symptoms and Affective Disorders

Major depressive episodes have as their essential feature either a dysphoric mood, usually depression, or loss of interest or pleasure in all or almost all usual activities or pastimes. (This disturbance is associated with other symptoms of depressive disorder as outlined in Chapter 4.) In many elderly depressed patients, paranoid delusions and hallucinations also occur. Their content is usually consistent with the dysphoric mood (mood congruent). Patients often feel that they are being persecuted because of sinfulness or some inadequacy. Other typical delusions include nihilistic delusions of world or personal destruction, hypochondriacal delusions of cancer or some other serious illness, or delusions of poverty. If hallucinations occur, they are usually simple and transient and may involve voices that criticize the patient for shortcomings. In rare instances, persecutory delusions in depression do not appear related to the mood disturbance and the patient is at a loss to explain why s/he is the object of persecution (mood incongruent).

In purely depressive and anxious-depressive states, many elderly people develop ideas of reference. The patient may feel that people are looking at him/her critically or talking about him/her in a derogatory way. If the depressive disorder is relatively mild, insight will be preserved and the patient will acknowledge the imaginary nature of those feelings. In more severe states, as noted, paranoid delusions and hallucinations with loss of insight may occur. In one series of elderly patients with depression, 38 percent exhibited paranoid features. It should also be noted that elderly hypomanic or manic patients may develop persecutory delusions with content derived from the patient's grandiose feeling of being envied or from attempts to restrain the patient's activities.

Finally affective symptoms may occur in paraphrenic illness. Among 93 patients with confirmed persistent persecutory disorders, 57 percent displayed some affective symptoms.

Recluses

Post (1980) has described a group of elderly patients who exhibit a very specific type of paranoid behavior as senile recluses. In these patients, increasing self-imposed social isolation results in deterioration of hygiene and self-care. Often they have withdrawn from all contacts with other people and may have barricaded themselves into their homes. Complaints from neighbors and/or health authorities often result in their being brought to treatment. In one study, 72 recluses were identified and an annual incidence rate of 6.5 cases per 1000 people over age 65 was reported. Widowed females predominated in the sample. Over one-half were diagnosed as psychotic including senile dementia with paranoid features, schizophrenia, paraphrenia, depression, and alcoholism. In some of these patients, rehabilitation in a day-hospital proved successful.

Paranoid Schizophrenia

Finally, it should be remembered that patients who develop schizophrenia early in life do grow old. As a result of deinstitutionalization, many elderly schizophrenic patients are living in the community. With increasing age, acute exacerbations of paranoid and other symptoms become less frequent and much lower dosages of antipsychotic medication are required to control symptoms. As noted previously, it has been observed that paranoid symptoms tend to disappear with chronicity in these patients. Often paranoid schizophrenic patients' most prominent symptom is schizophrenic thought disorder resulting in some degree of incoherence. It is important to distinguish these individuals from those suffering from dementia.

Also, there are a few patients who develop disorders displaying both affective and schizophrenic features late in life. Among schizophrenic features, delusions and/or hallucinations may be included. Schizo-affective patients are usually seen as occupying a mid-point between the schizophrenic and affective disorders rather than as suffering from a separate disease.

MANAGEMENT

Treatment of elderly patients with paranoid illnesses is usually effective if antipsychotic medication can be administered. Unfortunately, in too many cases this does not occur. It is extremely difficult to cultivate a supportive therapeutic relationship with a paranoid patient because of extreme suspicious-ness and lack of trust. The immediate treatment goal is to reduce the anxiety which underlies the paranoid ideas. This can be accomplished by three differing but related techniques: by psychotherapeutic intervention, by reducing the threat from the external environment and by anxiety-alleviating drugs (Busse and Pfeiffer 1977).

The first task in psychotherapeutic management is the establishment of a therapeutic alliance. At some point, the patient must ally with the therapist in a quest for relief from his/her suffering. With regard to delusions, it is important initially neither to agree with delusions nor to challenge them. In order to avoid arguments concerning the degree of truth in a delusion, the therapist should focus on how the delusion interferes with the patient's ability to carry on a normal life. This may lead to the identification of problems such as irritability, insomnia, or difficulty with concentration, but which the patient may be able to accept as hindrances with which the therapist might help. If possible, subjects such as hospitalization and medication should be avoided early on as paranoid patients are hypersensitive to restrictions of freedom. Only when some degree of agreement as to which problems will be dealt with has been reached, and some trust has been established, should these options be introduced. It is very important to be open and consistent with paranoid patients to enable the development of trust. The therapist must also learn to expect and tolerate anger and criticism and to advise patients that if they do grow suspicious of the therapist, they should not terminate the relationship. Both humor and inap-propriate reassurance should be avoided as paranoid patients often feel they are being made fun of, and they may consider the therapist who attempts to downplay the seriousness of their difficulties as naive and foolish. It is especially important for the therapist to be able to tolerate patients' overreactions. The goals of psychotherapeutic management are to restore the patient's self-esteem and to provide calm, empathic understanding of the patient's very frightening life situation. Once a relationship has developed, patients may be helped to consider alternative explanations for what they believe to be happening to them. Current life stresses and especially losses should be explored and empathy with regard to feelings of loss and vulnerability should be provided. Some shaping of behavior can be achieved if the therapist begins to attend selectively to reality-based information and concerns. In keeping with an emphasis on consistency, the patient should be reassured that the therapist's services will continue to be available to counteract fears of loss of control. If a supportive psychotherapeutic relationship can be established, confinement can often be avoided and treatment carried out without hospitalization.

Consideration must be given to many different types of environmental manipulation. Efforts must be made to correct sensory or cognitive deficits if they occur. Hearing aids and glasses should be supplied if indicated. Adequate lighting and sound levels should be assured. Homemaking services, if necessary, should be arranged. It is important to work with family members and neighbors towards the provision of a relatively stable, friendly, and familiar environment. Some elderly patients with relatively mild paranoid conditions may benefit from a change of environment. In general, however, stability, familiarity, and lack of complications should characterize the environment for paranoid patients. In keeping with the need for openness in establishing trust, it is always important to state very clearly what steps are to be taken and the purpose of each of these steps.

Antipsychotic medication is the most important treatment component for elderly patients suffering from moderate to severe paranoid conditions. It is important, of course, to identify the etiology of the paranoid symptoms. If symptoms are secondary to delirium or to depression, for example, then treatment of the underlying condition is essential. However, even in these situations, along with primary paranoid disorders and paranoid features arising in dementia, antipsychotic medication has a specific effect upon delusions and hallucinations. The problem, however, is that paranoid patients are suspicious of many things, including medication given to them. It has been reported that 60 percent of drug dosages given to paranoid patients in pill form are never taken. Patients may develop delusions about the medication itself, believing that it is poisonous or that the drugs cause people to talk about them. The best way to introduce medication is to suggest to the patient that s/he requires some assistance in dealing with the anxiety, irritability, and sleeplessness produced by the persecution, rather than by suggesting medication for delusions and hallucinations themselves. Again, in keeping with the necessity for openness and the development of trust, it is important to fully explore the patient's feelings about taking medications and to help work through resistance by explaining the indications, contraindications, and side effects of the medication.

Most elderly patients respond to small or only moderately large dosages of antipsychotic medication. Thioridazine, haloperidol, and loxapine are the drugs most frequently recommended. The choice will depend on whether the clinician is most concerned about anticholinergic effects such as drowsiness and hypotension or neurological effects such as parkinsonism and akathisia. No matter which antipsychotic drug is chosen, elderly patients must be monitored carefully for signs of tardive dyskinesia.

Low daytime dosages with more substantial dosages given at night are effective and tend to minimize side effects. Recommended dosages of thioridazine are 25 mg three times daily plus 50 to 100 mg at bedtime or haloperidol 0.5 to 1.0 mg three times daily plus 1 to 2 mg at bedtime. Dosages should be low initially, building up to higher dosages each week over two or three weeks (e.g. thioridazine 50 mg daily the first week, 100 mg daily the second week, 200 mg daily the third week). Once hallucinations cease and delusional ideas are no longer voiced spontaneously, dosages should not be further increased. The same medication should be used for at least four weeks for an adequate trial. There is general agreement that medications should be administered to paranoid patients in liquid or concentrated form with fruit juice or other liquid, to assure that the patient receives the medication. (A protocol for prescribing major tranquillizers is presented in Chapter 11.)

An alternate drug strategy is to use depot injections of long-acting antipsychotic medication. This of course has the advantage of providing assurance that the drug is indeed in the patient's system. Drugs such as fluphenazine decanoate (Modecate) given every three to four weeks in very low dosages (6 mg) are often very effective in these patients. Usually two or three injections are required before full remission is achieved. One month after remission has been achieved with antipsychotic medication, the lowest drug dosage on which the patient remains symptom-free should be determined. Yearly attempts should be made to withdraw antipsychotic medication to avoid the development of tardive dyskinesia.

With regard to prognosis, before the use of antipsychotic medication there had been a strong impression that the outlook was poor for elderly patients with paranoid disorders. In the absence of dementia, duration of life was not shortened but delusional beliefs persisted and some patients required ongoing hospital care. Now, however, with antipsychotic medication, treatment of elderly paraphrenics can be undertaken with a high expectation of success. In a 1966 study, 71 patients were treated with antipsychotic medications; 6 failed to respond completely; 22 continued to have delusional beliefs but the intensity of symptoms diminished to the point where discharge from hospital and successful reentry into the community was achieved; and 43 patients ceased to have ongoing symptoms. However, only about half of those 43 gained insight. On longer term follow-up, factors correlating with patient success included good response to the initial treatment episode, achievement of at least a modicum of insight, and patient and family co-operation with maintenance medication which itself was positively associated with the preservation of good relationships between the patient and significant others including the psychiatrist! Other characteristics associated with good, long-term outcome were relatively young age, being married, existing close relationship, mild rather than markedly deviant premorbid personality traits, relatively good sexual adjustment, and short duration of paranoid symptoms prior to treatment. Deafness and dementia were associated with poor outcome.

Currently, with a greater choice of medications and especially with the availability of depot preparations, failure of response should rarely occur and outcome for these patients is much improved.

REFERENCES AND SUGGESTED READINGS

American Psychiatric Association. 1980. *Diagnostic and Statistical Manual of Mental Disorders.* 3rd ed.

Busse E. W. and E. Pfeiffer. 1977. "Functional Psychiatric Disorders in Old Age." *Behavior and Adaptation in Late Life.* Ed. E. W. Busse and E. Pfeiffer. Boston: Little, Brown and Company.

Cooper A. F., A. R. Currey and D. W. K. Kay et al. 1974. "Hearing Loss in Paranoid and Affective Psychoses in the Elderly." *Lancet.* 2: 851.

Depare R. A. and C. Woodburn. 1975. "Disappearance of Paranoid Symptoms with Chronicity." *Journal of Abnormal Psychology.* 84: 84.

Kay D. W. K., A. F. Cooper and R. F. Garside et al. 1976. "The Differentiation of Paranoid from Affective Psychoses by Patients' Premorbid Characteristics." *British Journal of Psychiatry.* 129: 207.

Leuchter A. F. and J. E. Spar. 1985. "The Late-Onset Psychoses: Clinical and Diagnostic Features." *Journal of Nervous and Mental Diseases.* 173: 488.

Pfeiffer E. 1977. "Psychopathology and Social Pathology." *Handbook of the Psychology of Aging.* Ed. J. E. Birren and K. W. Schane. New York: Van Nostrand Rheinhold Company.

Post F. 1966. *Persistent Persecutory States of the Elderly.* England: Permagon Press Ltd.

Post F. 1973. "Paranoid Disorders in the Elderly." *Postgraduate Medicine.* 53: 52.

Post F. 1980. "Paranoid, Schizophrenia-like and Schizophrenic States in the Aged." *Handbook of Mental Health and Aging.* Ed. J. E. Birren and R. B. Sloane. Englewood Cliffs: Prentice-Hall Inc.

Retterstol N. 1968. "Paranoid Psychoses." *British Journal of Psychiatry.* 114: 533.

Retterstol N. 1970. *Prognosis in Paranoid Psychoses.* Springfield: Charles C. Thomas.

Roth M. 1955. "The Natural History of Mental Disorder in Old Age." *Journal of Mental Science.* 101: 281.

Shapiro D. 1965. *Neurotic Styles.* New York: Basic Books, Inc.

Sjogren H. 1964. "Paraphrenic, Melancholic and Psychoneurotic States in the Presenile-Senile Period of Life." *Acta Psychiatrica Scandinavica.* 176.

Slater E. and M. Roth (eds.) 1969. *Clinical Psychiatry.* London: Balliere, Tindall and Cassell.

8

Substance Abuse

Lynda A. Perry, M.S.W., C.S.W.

Substance abuse refers to a harmful dependence on or excessive use of any substance. The term typically is used in connection with heavy alcohol consumption and illicit drug usage. However, substance abuse is a broader term which encompasses more than alcoholism or drug addiction. The term can be used to describe excessive or inappropriate use of any substance including prescription drugs and over-the-counter medication.

FREQUENCY AND DISTRIBUTION

The prevalence of substance abuse in the elderly population is difficult to determine precisely. There is evidence that the problem has been under-recognized and under-reported in the past for a variety of reasons. These reasons include a general lack of interest in this age group, an unwillingness to consider grandparent figures as alcoholics, symptoms being mistakenly attributed to other causes such as advanced age, and the social isolation of the elderly which allows the problem to be less visible.

It is becoming clearer, however, that the elderly abuse alcohol at about the same rate as any other age group, that is, about 5 to 7 percent of people age 60 and over are alcoholics. In institutional settings this rate goes up to approximately 20 percent and in veterans' facilities it may reach as high as 40 percent. The rate of alcohol consumption may well be lower in volume in the older population but deleterious effects are still evident.

With respect to drug abuse, the prevalence figures are even less clear. The present geriatric population is comprised of a generation which were not inclined to use illegal drugs when they were young. Therefore, it is not surprising that the prevalence of illicit drug use in later years is also low. This problem may increase as today's younger generation ages.

The elderly consume large quantities of prescription and over-the-counter medications. In the United States, the elderly receive two and a half times more prescriptions than their proportion in the population would predict, and 80 percent of those prescriptions are for mood-altering substances. The average older person has been found to take four medications each day including both over-the-counter and prescription medications. While this high usage is partially accounted for by the elderly having more medical problems, it is likely that some of the consumption is abusive and based on harmful dependencies rather than therapeutic necessity. (Polypharmacy or multiple drug use in general is described in Chapter 11.)

DEFINITION OF SUBSTANCE ABUSE

It is difficult to define the dividing line between normal or heavy use and the abuse of a substance. It is not simply a matter of quantity in many cases. For example, one person has an average of three drinks each day and is considered to be a social drinker. Another person has an alcohol problem and yet also averages three drinks per day. The difference is in the impact which the alcohol has on one's body and on one's life. One person may have a glass of wine with lunch and dinner regularly and a drink or two in the evening. These three drinks are spaced well apart in time and consumed with food thus allowing the body to metabolize the alcohol before it reaches toxic levels. The other person may not drink everyday but rather consumes 21 drinks per week on one or two days becoming quite intoxicated and incapable of adequately performing ordinary taks. His/her behavior when intoxicated may be jeopardizing marriage and family relationships. A third person may have a drinking pattern similar to the first, but because of a different body metabolism may be suffering toxic effects.

The Diagnostic and Statistical Manual of Mental Disorders, Third Edition (*DSM-III*) uses a three level typology in describing substance abuse (see Table 8.1). The first level is described as recreational use or occasional intoxication without a pattern of pathological use. The next level is termed abuse and involves a pattern of pathological use coupled with impairment in social or occupational functioning which has been occurring for at least one month. A pattern of pathological abuse is defined somewhat differently depending on the substance being abused but in each case involves daily use and an inability to decrease or cease usage.

TABLE 8.1

305.0 Alcohol Abuse

Differential diagnosis. Nonpathological recreational use of a substance, episodes of intoxication without a pattern of pathological use.

Diagnostic Criteria

A. *Pattern of pathological alcohol use:* need for daily use of alcohol for adequate functioning; inability to cut down or stop drinking; repeated efforts to control or reduce excess drinking by "going on the wagon" (periods of temporary abstinence) or restricting drinking to certain times of the day; binges (remaining intoxicated throughout the day for at least two days); occasional consumption of a fifth of spirits (or its equivalent in wine or beer); amnesic periods for events occurring while intoxicated (blackouts); continuation of drinking despite a serious physical disorder that the individual knows is exacerbated by alcohol use; drinking of non-beverage alcohol.

B. *Impairment in social or occupational functioning due to alcohol use:* e.g., violence while intoxicated, absence from work, loss of job, legal difficulties (e.g., arrest for intoxicated behaviour, traffic accidents while intoxicated), arguments or difficulties with family or friends because of excessive alcohol use.

C. *Duration of disturbance of at least one month.*

305.4 Barbiturate or Similarly Acting Sedative or Hypnotic Abuse

Diagnostic criteria

A. *Pattern of pathological use:* inability to cut down or stop use; intoxication throughout the day; frequent use of the equivalent of 600 mg or more of secobarbital or 60 mg or more of intoxicant.

B. *Impairment in social or occupational functioning due to substance use:* e.g., fights, loss of friends, absence from work, loss of job, or legal difficulties (other than a single arrest due to possession, purchase or sale of the substance).

C. Duration of disturbance of at least one month.

American Psychiatric Association Diagnostic and Statistical Manual of Mental Disorders, Third Edition. Washington, DC, copyright APA 1980. Used with permission.

The third level described in *DSM-III* is termed dependence. This diagnosis requires either tolerance or withdrawal. Tolerance is defined as the "need for markedly increased amounts of the substance to achieve the desired effect, or markedly diminished effect with regular use of the same amount" (*DSM-III*). Withdrawal refers to the appearance of withdrawal symptoms after cessation or reduction of use. Withdrawal symptoms include: nausea and vomiting, malaise or weakness, rapid heart beat, sweating, high blood pressure, anxiety, depressed mood or irritability, tremors, and orthostatic hypotension.

TABLE 8.2

303.9 Alcohol Dependence

Diagnostic Criteria

A. Either a pattern of pathological use or impairment in social or occupational functioning due to alcohol use.

Pattern of pathological alcohol use: daily use of alcohol is a prerequisite for adequate functioning; inability to cut down or stop drinking; repeated efforts to control or reduce excess drinking by "going on the wagon" (periods of temporary abstinence) or restriction of drinking to certain times of the day; drinks non-beverage alcohol; goes on binges (remains intoxicated throughout the day for at least two days); occasionally drinks a fifth of spirits (or its equivalent in wine or beer); has had two or more "blackouts" (amnesic period for events occurring while intoxicated); continues to drink despite a serious physical disorder that the individual knows is exacerbated by alcohol use.

Impairment in social or occupational functioning due to alcohol use: e.g., violence while intoxicated, absence from work, loss of job, legal difficulties (e.g., arrest for intoxicated behavior, traffic accidents while intoxicated), arguments or difficulties with family or friends because of excessive alcohol use.

B. Either tolerance or withdrawal:

(1) *Tolerance*: need for markedly increased amounts of alcohol to achieve the desired effect, or markedly diminished effects with regular use of the same amount.

(2) *Withdrawal*: development of alcohol withdrawal (e.g., morning "shakes" and malaise relieved by drinking) after cessation of or reduction in drinking.

304.1 Barbiturate or Similarly Acting Sedative or Hypnotic Dependence

---

Diagnostic criteria

Either tolerance or withdrawal.

Tolerance: need for markedly increased amounts of the substance to achieve the desired effect, or markedly diminished effect with regular use of the same amount.

Withdrawal: development of barbiturate or similarly acting sedative or hypnotic withdrawal after cessation of or reduction in substance use.

American Psychiatric Association Diagnostic and Statistical Manual of Mental Disorders, Third Edition. Washington, DC, copyright APA 1980. Used with permission.

ABUSE OF PRESCRIPTION AND OVER-THE-COUNTER MEDICATIONS

Non-compliance with regimens of prescription medications occurs frequently. (Many of the factors contributing to non-compliance, as well as the principles to be followed to increase compliance, are discussed in Chapter 11.) Non-compliance in the form of taking more medication than prescribed may be indicative of a harmful dependence. Similarly, the use of a medication for a reason other than that for which it was prescribed may indicate possible abuse.

Psychotropic medications (e.g. sleeping pills and tranquillizers), analgesics (pain killers), and antihistamines (e.g. nasal decongestants), are particularly susceptible to being abused. These medications have properties which alter perception of pain or discomfort and which may produce a euphoric state which is pleasant to some people. After a period of usage of these medications, a person may begin to fear that s/he is unable to cope with life without the drug. When this occurs, a form of psychological dependency has been created.

There is a physical component to the dependency in some cases. The rebound effect describes the condition wherein discontinuation of a medication results in a strong return of the original symptom. For example, some of the benzodiazepines (Valium, Vivol, etc.) produce a change in the sleep cycle. When a person has taken diazepam regularly and then stops, s/he frequently experiences a rebound effect and has more trouble sleeping than before taking the medication. Antihistamines, particularly in the form of nasal sprays, also produce a rebound effect.

Many drugs such as barbiturates, benzodiazepines, alcohol, opiates, and amphetamines may produce very unpleasant and potentially dangerous symptoms when prolonged heavy use is reduced or discontinued. The appearance of these symptoms is often a driving factor in continued use and abuse even when the person wishes to stop the dependence.

Many dependencies on prescribed medications begin quite innocently when a medication is appropriately prescribed for a genuine symptom and taken as directed for a period of time. The problem may begin when the physician does not monitor the patient completely in order to decrease and eventually to discontinue the medication at the appropriate time. Alternately, the patient may continue to request the medication (perhaps from several doctors) after being told it is time to reduce the dosage or to discontinue its use. Over-the-counter preparations may be substituted if a prescription is not available.

Medications may be prescribed in excessive dosages or without sufficient indication of requirement. In these cases, the abuse of the drug is almost completely iatrogenic. This is quite commonly encountered in patients complaining of insomnia. (This issue is addressed in some detail in Chapter 11.) Elderly patients complaining of a sleep disturbance should first be encouraged to try non-drug strategies to improve their sleep habits. Failing that, short acting hypnotics in dosages about one-half of the usually recommended adult dosage should be given a brief trial. In no case should barbiturates be prescribed because of their strong potential for inducing dependency and their lethality when taken in overdosage. Dependencies on over-the-counter preparations may include sedatives which are often abused by older people.

Some physicians may have difficulty firmly resisting the demands of some patients for dependency producing drugs. Some physicians may also hold the misguided belief that the dependency causes no harm. This attitude is especially prevalent in the treatment of the elderly who may be regarded as unproductive in any case, and therefore, not hampered by the effects of drugs. The reality is that older people, who are dependent on drugs which are not therapeutically necessary, are suffering from diminished quality of life. For example, the effects or side effects of the medications may be affecting their ability to think clearly and to control their emotions. Those medications may also be affecting their ability to walk unaided, to see clearly, or to control other aspects of their physical functioning.

ALCOHOL ABUSE

Elderly abusers of alcohol may have a long history of heavy alcohol consumption. They may have been alcoholic for years and continued the pattern into old age despite the effects on their bodies and lifestyle. It may be that their heavy consumption did not produce harmful effects when they were younger. The changing metabolism of old age (see also Chapter 1), with or without an increase in consumption, may create a drinking problem for a previously controlled drinker. Many of these long-time drinkers have a severe lack of social skills which become more prominent and problematic in retirement years.

Another group of elderly alcohol abusers were occasional or light drinkers through their adult years but became problem drinkers late in life. As with prescription drug abuse, alcohol abuse in this group may begin innocuously when a person uses alcohol in a socially acceptable manner to relax during a time of stress. The stress may be the transition to retirement or the death of a spouse. Problems begin when the use of alcohol becomes the predominant or the only coping mechanism and begins to have a negative impact on the person's physical well-being as well as on his/her lifestyle. Whether a person has been drinking heavily all his/her life or begins late in life, the harmful effects on the body are similar. Individuals who experience the onset of alcoholism later in life, quickly catch up in terms of impact on health.

Older alcohol abusers appear to be more susceptible to alcohol induced cognitive loss. In any age group, alcohol intoxication impairs brain cell function leading to memory loss, confusion, and disorientation. The cognitive functions usually do improve shortly after the alcohol has left the body. However, when a person has been drinking heavily over a long period of time, it may take several weeks or months of abstinence for the brain to regain its previous level of functioning. It is important to reassess periodically to determine whether abilities lost while drinking have been regained during abstinence.

Prolonged, heavy usage of alcohol can produce permanent brain damage. Korsakoff's syndrome and Wernicke's encephalopathy are most commonly caused by alcohol abuse and vitamin deficiency due to the malnutrition which is frequently secondary to that abuse. The hallmark of Korsakoff's syndrome is confabulation which is the tendency to fill in gaps of memory with detailed and plausible but incorrect responses. The memory loss is usually permanent. Patients with Wernicke's encephalopathy present with delirium, ataxia (impaired gait), and decreased eye movements. Patients usually recover with appropriate treatment but may be left with residual symptoms of Korsakoff's syndrome.

Other harmful effects caused by alcohol abuse include damage to the liver, injuries due to accidents and falls, malnutrition, poor family relationships, and financial difficulties. Presence of these medical and social indicators in a client's history should trigger suspicion of possible alcohol abuse.

Liver disease is common in alcoholics because of the way alcohol is metabolized by the body. Heavy alcohol consumption leads to fat accumulation in the liver and reduced liver function. Some of the engorged cells may die and produce an inflammation characteristic of alcoholic hepatitis. Further drinking leads to more dead liver cells, increased inflammation and the development of scar tissue in the liver—the hallmark of cirrhosis. The continuing poor functioning of the diseased liver can result in a number of serious consequences including hepatic coma and death.

Injuries due to accidents are common in alcohol abusers. Falls are the most common cause of accidental death in the elderly. The unsteady gait, poor motor control, and impaired judgment all associated with alcohol intoxication, make the alcohol abuser a prime candidate for falls and other accidents.

Fires are frequently caused by a person lapsing into a deep sleep due to heavy alcohol consumption and leaving a cigarette or a pot burning on the stove. The alcoholic is often unable to satisfactorily account for the accident due to memory loss and perhaps the defence mechanism of denial.

Malnutrition is often secondary to alcohol abuse because the caloric content of alcohol depresses hunger. The heavy drinker will frequently forgo food in favor of alcohol. In addition, alcohol itself enhances malnutrition by impairing digestion of food and the absorption of nutrients by the body.

Poor family relationships are common in the families of alcoholics. Long-time alcoholics may have lost contact with family members years ago. Children may feel unable to offer support to the parent who did not support them when they were young. Even the late onset alcoholic may have alienated family by rebuffing offers of help. Families of alcoholics need a great deal of support to be useful resources in the treatment program.

Financial difficulties are common because the cost involved in heavy alcohol consumption frequently leads to unpaid bills. Also, poor judgment while intoxicated may lead to frivolous spending, high car insurance rates, and poor money management. Prolonged and heavy substance abuse can thus have a very harmful effect on an individual's biological and social functioning.

SUBSTANCE ABUSE AND OTHER MENTAL DISORDERS

Alcohol and Depression

Depression is the most common mental disorder. (See also Chapter 4.) Its symptoms of feeling down, irritable, hopeless, and helpless motivate the sufferer to seek relief. Alcohol is a readily available mood-altering drug and is therefore frequently used by people suffering from depression in an effort to alleviate their symptoms. Unfortunately, alcohol itself has a depressant effect and thus only enhances the depression.

If the individual continues to use alcohol, the drinking itself may become a serious problem which has to be controlled before help can be found for the underlying depression. It is considered unwise to give antidepressant medications to anyone using alcohol heavily. The interaction of the medication with alcohol produces uncertain effects. Also, the potential for a suicide attempt must be seriously considered with a depressed alcoholic who is likely to be lacking in impulse control.

Alcohol and Paranoia

In some individuals, alcohol abuse leads to the development of paranoid ideas. Unfounded and unshakable jealousy is one form of paranoid thinking to which alcoholics are susceptible.

Alcohol and Delirium

Intoxication with alcohol or other drugs is in fact a form of delirium (which is discussed in detail in Chapter 6). The symptoms of delirium include a clouding of consciousness, disorientation, slurred speech, impaired memory, and impaired judgment. The delirium caused by intoxication will generally subside as the body metabolizes and excretes the substance. However, delirium is a potentially serious medical condition and should be properly assessed and treated.

Delirium tremens (DTs) which is a common symptom of alcohol withdrawal can progress to coma and death. Early symptoms include restlessness, slight confusion and visual illusions and hallucinations.

Alcoholic and other substance abusers are at risk for delirium caused by other factors also, such as, infections and drug side effects. The brain damage caused by chronic substance abuse results in increased susceptibility to delirium whenever the flow of oxygen to the brain is decreased. The potentially serious consequences of delirium dictate the importance of early recognition, accurate diagnosis, and effective treatment.

DIAGNOSING SUBSTANCE ABUSE

Recognizing substance abusers requires an awareness of the harmful effects described earlier because frequently individuals do not seek help for their substance abuse but present with symptoms caused by the abuse. An older person showing symptoms of intoxication may not be recognized as alcoholic because the unsteady gait, slurred speech, and confusion may be erroneously attributed to other ailments. It is useful to maintain an index of suspicion regarding substance abuse and to inquire about use of alcohol, prescription drugs, caffeine, and over-the-counter preparations as part of the standard intake assessment.

This assessment should include questions regarding whether the person uses or has used any of these substances. A negative response would be followed by some probing about how the individual handles situations in which use of one of these substances is common. For example, inquiring about headaches and sleeplessness, may elicit information about over-the-counter preparations. A complete list of medications, their dosages, how often they are taken, how long they have been taken, and the individual's understanding of their purpose is part of a standard assessment. The response to these questions may alert the interviewer to the possibility of abuse. Seeing the vials allows the interviewer to determine whether more than one doctor and/or pharmacy are supplying the medications. In the case of a clinic or group practice, more than one physician may legitimately have prescribed medication..

The inquiry into use of alcohol, cigarettes, and caffeine follows a similar pattern. The amount and frequency of use, the history of use, and of any attempts to stop usage are important questions. In addition, questions regarding possible effects of heavy alcohol consumption include inquiry about blackouts as well as the medical and social indicators outlined previously. Questions about use of leisure time, friendships, and family relationships will also provide clues to the existence of substance abuse. A review of the diagnostic criteria outlined in Table 8.1 will provide suggestions for relevant inquiry. (See also Chapter 9 which provides guidelines for a full clinical assessment.)

It is important to ask questions in a matter-of-fact, non-judgmental manner. Substance abusers tend to have a low self-esteem and are very sensitive to criticism implied by tone of voice and body language.

Home visits can be very useful in recognizing those substances abusers who may present well during an office assessment. The homes of substance abusers are often poorly maintained and may show evidence of cigarette burns or other small fires. Abusers of medications frequently have large quantities of pill bottles and preparations in every room. They may even have several brands of similar medications. These indicators are not proof of substance abuse, but rather suggest the possibility. The clinician needs to explore each physical or social indicator to determine whether it is due to substance abuse. It is usually necessary to interview other family members, friends, or involved social agencies to achieve an accurate description of substance abuse patterns.

MANAGEMENT

A frequent difficulty in working with substance abusers is arriving at a mutually agreed upon definition of a problem and a wish to make a change. It is not necessary, and may be counter-productive with seniors, to insist upon labelling the substance abuse as the chief problem. If one or more of the harmful effects can be identified as a problem which the client would like to resolve, the stage is set to gradually identify the abuse as something which will have to change in order to solve the problem.

One of the challenges of working with substance abusers is assisting them to strengthen their sense of competence so they do not feel overwhelmed as they begin to recognize the extent of their problems. Bolstering self-esteem by giving them honest praise at every opportunity is required to enhance clients' sense of mastery and control. These will be important resources as the clients work to eliminate or decrease their dependence on alcohol or drugs.

Counselling should be directed towards improving social skills and finding interesting and pleasurable activities to use time more effectively. Practical counselling focussed on problem-solving techniques and improved self-care will generally be more useful than insight-oriented psychotherapy with this population. Specific assistance, such as a homemaker to help the client improve home surroundings, may be necessary in the early stages when the client may be overwhelmed and immobilized by the extent of his/her problems.

Alcoholics Anonymous has achieved the best results in helping people recover from alcoholism. Peer support combined with positive thinking techniques form the foundation of an AA program. Clients should be encouraged and assisted to attend AA meetings. Al Anon may be helpful for the relatives of alcoholics whether or not the drinker is seeking help.

Building trust may be very slow when working with the elderly alcoholic. It is often necessary to make several home visits before being able to involve the client in a treatment program. Once some level of trust has been established, a crisis such as a fire, an eviction notice, or a medical emergency can be utilized effectively to help the client recognize the harmful effects of the substance abuse. A few days later, a rationalization may have been developed. At the time of the crisis the client may be willing to acknowledge the problem and begin to plan for change.

In some cases, medical supervision is necessary to manage the early detoxification stage while the client decreases or discontinues use of drugs or alcohol. It is particularly important that barbiturates not be discontinued without medical supervision because of the risk of seizures during withdrawal.

CONCLUSION

Abusive use of alcohol, prescription drugs, and over-the-counter preparations are frequently encountered in the older population. The health care professional must be alert to this possibility and aware of medical and social indicators suggestive of problems in the area of substance abuse.

Treatment of elderly substance abusers involves enhancing the client's sense of competence, focussing on practical issues, and assisting in the development of a support network.

REFERENCES AND SUGGESTED READINGS

American Psychiatric Association. 1980. *Diagnostic and Statistical Manual of Mental Disorders.* 3rd ed.

Caroselli-Karinja Marie. June 1985. "Drug Abuse and the Elderly." *Journal of Psychosocial Nursing.* 23: 25–28.

Dobbie Judy. Fall 1977. "Substance Abuse Among the Elderly." *Addictions.*

Lieber Charles S. March 1976. "The Metabolism of Alcohol. *Scientific American.* 234: 25–34.

Lishman W. A. 1981. "Cerebral Disorder in Alcoholism—Syndromes of Impairment." *Brain.* 104: 1–20.

Schuckit Marc A., Elizabeth R. Morrissey and R. Michael O'Leary. 1978. "Alcohol Problems in Elderly Men and Women." *Addictive Diseases: An International Journal.* 3: 405–416.

Zimberg Sheldon. 1978. "Treatment of the Elderly Alcoholic in the Community and In An Institutional Setting." *Addictive Diseases: An International Journal.* 3: 417–427.

Part Three
ASSESSMENT AND MANAGEMENT

9

Clinical Assessment

Barry A. Martin, M.D., F.R.C.P. (C)

The clinical assessment of geriatric patients includes all those observations necessary to plan appropriate treatment and management of their presenting problems. The essential elements of a full inquiry and investigation include the history, physical and mental status examinations, assessments of activities of daily living and financial competence, and ancillary clinical and laboratory tests as required.

The examination of elderly patients may be complicated by the presence of primary sensory deficits and other physical disabilities. Furthermore, some of the specific symptoms of functional and organic mental disorders directly interfere with the acquisition of accurate information. The assessment procedures must be adapted to offset these problems.

The principal objective of the assessment is to reach an accurate diagnosis. The application of a psychiatric diagnosis to a patient's symptoms or behavior implies that a certain level or threshold of severity has been reached. This diagnostic decision is an important initial step to mitigate the unnecessary treatment of benign symptoms of self-limiting problems. An accurate diagnosis is also necessary to prescribe specific treatment or, if none is available, to give a prognosis of the natural history of the disorder. The definition of appropriate objectives for social and rehabilitation programs is also dependent, in large part, upon the patient's diagnosis and prognosis. Thus, the psychiatric diagnosis provides the overall conceptual framework for case management. It should be noted that many diverse observations of a patient's behavior are often necessary to make and/or confirm a diagnosis. If made by a reliable witness, they are valuable components of the assessment. Therefore, the members of all clinical disciplines should attempt to make and record complete and accurate observations.

This chapter summarizes the general principles to be followed in conducting clinical interviews of geriatric patients. The salient features of a psychiatric history and mental status examination are described. The clinical examination for the major symptoms of depression and dementia is presented in detail.

THE CLINICAL INTERVIEW

Time and Setting

Insofar as possible, the circumstances of the examination should be conducive to obtaining accurate information. Reasonable attempts should be made to minimize any physical discomfort experienced by the patient and the interview should be interrupted when necessary to attend to such discomfort. When feasible, undue fatigue should be avoided by scheduling two or more interviews instead of one lasting more than an hour. If the patient is hungry, the interview should not extend well into the time for a scheduled meal.

To ensure privacy and confidentiality, the patient should be interviewed alone whenever possible. It is not satisfactory to conduct a psychiatric interview in an institution in a multiple-occupancy room with the curtains drawn around the patient's bed. If another person is to be present (as an informant, witness, or interpreter), it should be with the patient's permission.

Environmental distractions should be minimized (i.e. turn off the radio or television). The room must be illuminated adequately and any hearing impairment must be overcome. The examiner's speech should be slow, clear, and loud enough to be both comprehensible and comfortable to the patient. A voice amplifier should be used if necessary.

Therapeutic Relationship

There are two principal objectives of the clinical assessment interview—to obtain sufficient information to make a diagnosis and/or a management plan and to establish a therapeutic relationship with the patient. The relative emphasis on these two objectives will vary but rapport with the patient should not be jeopardized in the relentless pursuit of information.

The examiner and the purpose of the interview should be identified correctly to the patient. The psychiatric orientation of the assessment should not be disguised and the patient's apprehension or hostility should be addressed openly. The role of any other person in attendance must be clarified for the patient.

It must be remembered that much of the important information being sought in a psychiatric assessment may be quite inaccessible to both the examiner and the patient, for a number of reasons. Mental phenomena experienced by the patient are not directly observable for the most part except insofar as they influence behavior. The patient may be quite reluctant to discuss sensitive issues or to reveal embarrassing information. (Just the acknowledgment of symptoms of a mental disorder is often very embarrassing.) That reluctance must be acknowledged and respected. Tactful but forthright questions should be used to explore for potentially sensitive subject matter. The patient can be asked to identify troublesome issues with the assurance that they need not be discussed in detail. Later in the interview, the patient may be more comfortable or more trusting of the examiner and the subjects should be broached with the suggestion that further discussion may help to identify the sources of the problems. The examiner must be non-judgmental and comfortable with the issues in order to put the patient sufficiently at ease.

Many of the symptoms of mental disorders are very difficult to articulate. Many patients simply do not have the vocabulary to describe complex mental phenomena which, by definition, may be well beyond the range of normal experience. On the other hand, some symptoms (i.e. depressed mood and anxiety) are on a continuum with normal experience and it may be difficult to identify when the patient's own norm has been exceeded. Other experiences may not be identified as symptoms because they are mistakenly equated with ageing. Some patients may be unable or unwilling to describe emotional experiences in anything but physical terms such that the history consists largely of multiple somatic complaints. The interviewer must phrase and rephrase questions to suit the patient's vocabulary, to provide verbal cues with which the patient can identify his/her experiences, and to separate emotional from physical symptoms.

The interview should be conducted with a mixture of open and specific questions in order to establish and maintain rapport and to increase the accessibility of the patient's symptoms.

Informants

As a general rule, ancillary and corroborating information should be obtained from relatives or others in close association with the patient. Of course, this is essential in the presence of significant cognitive impairment. Informants may be able to describe the premorbid functioning of the patient and to identify when that began to deteriorate.

THE PSYCHIATRIC HISTORY

What follows is a summary of the format for taking a psychiatric history. An attempt should be made to obtain the information described under each heading in order to appreciate the many factors that may be contributing to the patient's presenting problems. There is very wide individual variation in the amount of pertinent information that can be and should be obtained under the various headings of the history. The general principles of interviewing, previously noted, should be applied in taking the history.

Identifying and Demographic Information

The interview should begin with the collection of basic descriptive information, which is emotionally quite "neutral", to give the patient time to become comfortable with the interviewer. As a suggested guideline, this information may include the following: full name and maiden name; age,

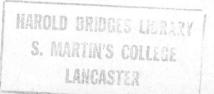

birthdate, birthplace; present address, previous address and date of move; highest education achieved; present or former occupation; marital status; name, age (or date of death) of spouse if applicable; names, ages, and occupations of children if applicable; and, dates of admissions to hospital (for physical and mental illness).

This synopsis of the patient's life rapidly orientates the examiner to the patient's present circumstances and ability to provide a reliable history. Substantial difficulty encountered in obtaining this information should alert the interviewer to the possibility of impaired cognitive function which should then be assessed early in the interview. (There is no point in pursuing a detailed history if the patient's memory is seriously impaired.)

Presenting Problems

The patient and/or informants should be asked to identify all of the reasons for the assessment. It is also useful to clarify what may have precipitated the assessment so that any immediate life crisis may be addressed.

History of Present Illness

The patient and/or informants should then be given the opportunity to describe the presenting problems. Very direct and specific questions should be used as necessary to clarify the description of the presenting symptoms and behavior, the date of onset, apparent precipitants, and subsequent course (i.e. fluctuations in the presence, duration, and severity of each symptom). It is important to identify events indicating a real or symbolic loss which are associated in time with the onset of the presenting problems.

The interviewer should form a preliminary impression of which major diagnostic category or categories (i.e. dementia, depression, paranoid disorder) may describe the patient's condition. The objective is then to obtain sufficient information about the presenting and related symptoms to confirm or refute that diagnostic impression. Therefore, specific inquiry must be made of the presence or absence of all the symptoms of the suspected disorder(s) in order to describe the complete clinical picture. [For example, a patient presents with the following symptoms: suspiciousness and distrust of other people, including the vaguely described belief that someone has been stealing his personal possessions; irritability and verbal abuse of his spouse; insomnia; decreased concentration; and, decreased interest in his usual activities with resultant social withdrawal. He has some difficulty remembering or is angrily dismissive of questions asked in order to obtain identifying and demographic information. Diagnoses of both dementia and depression should be entertained. In order to substantiate this impression, the interviewer must confirm the presence or absence of all the other major symptoms of these disorders. A suggested line of inquiry to be followed is presented in sections later in this chapter.]

It is preferable to flesh out the clinical picture or syndrome at this stage of the history while the patient's attention is focussed on the presenting symptoms. Some examiners prefer to leave the assessment of cognitive function to the end of the interview. However, a strong impression of cognitive impairment should be confirmed early in the interview because it will influence the content of the subsequent history.

It should be noted that this is the most important part of the history. The principal objective of the assessment is to make a diagnosis. An inadequate description of the presenting syndrome may undermine this objective. The remaining sections of the history provide information that confirms the diagnosis and/or which identifies issues to be addressed in an overall case management plan.

Past Psychiatric History

It is important to obtain any history of previous occurrences of the presenting problems in order to document the presence of a remitting and relapsing mental disorder. Details of all previous in- and out-patient treatment/consultations for emotional problems should be recorded. (As a general rule, discharge summaries of previous treatments should be obtained.)

Family and Marital History

This part of the history should concentrate primarily upon the patient's current circumstances. A brief overview of family life from childhood to the present should be obtained to identify the major sources of distress, including the deaths of parents and/or other family members. The extent of the bereavement following significant losses should be noted.

The marital relationship, including present sexual functioning, should be assessed to identify both long-standing conflict and the extent to which the presenting problems have interfered with the relationship.

The relationship to other family members, including children, siblings, and surviving parents, should be assessed. It may be instructive to learn how other family members have dealt with the problems of ageing and, specifically, to acquire an impression of how the patient's own parents aged. It is also important to assess the role of each family member in the present care of the patient and to form an impression of the burden created by that caregiving role.

In the context of family relationships, the patient's premorbid personality should be described. The extent to which that personality has changed during the course of the presenting problems should also be documented. Informants who are related to the patient may be best able to provide this information.

Educational and Occupational History

It is helpful to form an impression of the patient's premorbid intellectual capacity and skills with which to compare the present cognitive function. Therefore, educational accomplishments and job descriptions should be obtained. The degree of satisfaction derived from the lifetime employment should be assessed as well as the response to retirement. If work was the single most important activity, the patient's adaptation to retirement should be examined closely.

Social and Functional Capacity

The extent to which the presenting problems and/or premorbid personality or other disabilities may have interfered with activities of daily living should be assessed. This is best done by itemizing and describing the patient's usual activities and abilities under the following categories: self-maintenance (i.e. dressing and grooming, bathing and toiletting, nutrition, mobility); safety (i.e. smoking and cooking, hot water temperature, drug taking, motor vehicle operation); social network and use of support services; social and recreational activities; and financial competence.

Medical History

The past medical and surgical history should be summarized. All present physical disorders should be noted along with the current treatment. A detailed medication history should be taken including prescription and non-prescription drugs, alcohol and tobacco. (See also Chapter 11.)

THE MENTAL STATUS EXAMINATION

The mental status is the description of the patient's psychological/emotional state and cognitive functioning as observed during the assessment interview. It includes those symptoms uncovered while taking the history of the present illness and observations made throughout the interview.

The mental status examination is completed at the end of the assessment interview through inquiry about all pertinent symptoms that have not been addressed earlier. As previously noted, the examination of cognitive function may be left until the end of the interview if significant cognitive impairment is not suspected.

Observations are usually recorded under the following headings: appearance and behavior, speech, affect, thought form and content, perception, and cognitive function. Some of the observations and symptoms included in each are summarized in Table 9.1.

THE EXAMINATION FOR DEPRESSION

The clinical syndrome of depression is described in detail in Chapter 4 and the cardinal symptoms of depression are summarized in Table 9.2. In order to accurately diagnose the disorder and to estimate its severity, including the risk of suicide, the assessment should include determination of the presence or absence of each of those symptoms. Furthermore, each symptom has its own range or continuum of severity which is a measure of its clinical significance. Therefore, the severity of each symptom present should be assessed. Suggested guidelines and examples of questions for the clinical examination of some of the specific symptoms of depression are presented in the ensuing sections.

TABLE 9.1
The Mental Status Examination

1. **Appearance and Behavior**
    i.   Manner of relating to the interviewer
    ii. Appropriateness to the interview
    iii. Gross neglect of hygiene and grooming
    iv. Inanition and dehydration
    v.   Mobility
    vi. Bizarre behavior

2. **Speech**
    i.   Rate and articulation
    ii. Vocabulary (command of English)

3. **Affect**
    i.   Subjective and objective mood
    ii. Self-esteem
    iii. Future orientation
    iv. Suicidal ideation

4. **Thought Form and Content**
    i.   Coherence and logic
    ii. Themes with which the patient is preoccupied
    iii. Obsessional thoughts
    iv. Delusions

5. **Perception**
    i.   Illusions
    ii. Hallucinations
    iii. Depersonalization/derealization

6. **Cognitive Function**
    i.   Level of consciousness
    ii.   Orientation
    iii. Memory
    iv.   Attention and concentration
    v.   Language
    vi.   Visual-spatial organization
    vii. Abstract thinking
    viii. Judgment
    ix.   Insight

In keeping with recommendations presented earlier in this chapter, the line of inquiry and specific questions must be tailored to meet the clinical circumstances. Questions and/or instructions must be understood by the patient and phrased to maintain rapport. (In the following sections, examples of questions and instructions to the patient are italicized.)

TABLE 9.2

The Symptoms of Depression

1. Dysphoric mood; loss of interest or pleasure (anhedonia)
2. Diminished self-esteem: feelings of inadequacy, self-reproach, excessive or inappropriate guilt, feelings of uselessness or worthlessness
3. Decreased future orientation: pessimism, hopelessness
4. Suicidal ideation: diminished value of life, recurrent thoughts of death, wishes to be dead, thoughts of suicide, suicide plans, suicide attempt
5. Delusions: content congruent with the above-noted thoughts and feelings
6. Paranoid symptoms: ideas of reference; persecutory delusions (See Chapter 7.)
7. Depressive stupor: mute and unresponsive
8. Decreased ability to think clearly or concentrate; indecisiveness
9. Psychomotor agitation or retardation
10. Insomnia or hypersomnia: early morning awakening
11. Decreased sexual drive
12. Loss of energy; fatigue
13. Anorexia and significant weight loss or dehydration; increased appetite and significant weight gain
14. Somatic complaints: hypochondriasis

Dysphoric Mood and Anhedonia

The subjective mood experienced by patients with depression includes feelings of dissatisfaction and discontent, irritability and anger, anxiety, dread of the day, and pervasive sadness. The subjective experience of sadness may be underreported or denied by many geriatric patients. Therefore, the initial question should be phrased in general terms without suggesting a specific affective state. *How are you feeling lately? How have your spirits been?* If this does not elicit a response, then questions can be phrased to offer alternative responses. *Have you been in a good mood or feeling down and sad? Are you generally calm and relaxed or have you been getting tense and irritable or angry? Do you look forward to the day or do you wake up feeling terrible?* Leading or suggestive questions should not be used initially since the patient may just nod in assent. However, such questions should be used if the preceding inquiry is met with denial or vague responses. *Would the term "depressed" apply to the way you feel?* The patient should be asked to describe his/her experience in terms of frequency, duration, and severity (as compared to the normal mood and any similar experiences in the past). Diurnal variation should be assessed. *Is there any time of day when you feel at your worst? At your best?* The responsiveness of the mood to external events should be assessed. *What makes you feel better or worse?*

A more accessible measure or index of the severity of a dysphoric mood is the extent to which a patient has lost interest or pleasure in usual activities and personal relationships. Behaviorally, this may be reported as varying degrees of social withdrawal, work inhibition, and decreased productivity. The patient may also describe being unable to feel or being emotionally paralyzed or empty. It may be noticed as a distressing lack of empathy for someone close who is grieving. Again, inquiry should be initiated with general questions. *Have you kept up your usual interests in people and activities? Are you enjoying things as much as usual?* As a rule, an unqualified affirmative or negative response should not be accepted. Therefore, it is useful to quantify the activities and to identify recent changes. *Could you describe the activities which you enjoy? When was the last time you did that? That seems like quite some time ago— why haven't you been doing it lately?* Having identified a change in frequency or cessation of an activity, the patient may then be able to describe the associated feeling state. This change in activity may be temporally associated with the onset of depression. Anhedonia, the complete absence of pleasure in living, should be documented if present. *Is there nothing at all which you enjoy? Is there anyone you see or think about who makes you feel a little better?*

Diminished Self-esteem

Clinically significant depression is invariably accompanied by some diminution of the patient's self-esteem. This symptom distinguishes the mental disorder of depression from more transient and/or normal experiences of sadness or ennui which are attributed to external events or blamed on others. There is a very wide range of impairment of self-esteem in depression and it may be experienced by the patient in many ways, including the following: feelings of inadequacy or loss of confidence; self-reproach to self-loathing; excessive or inappropriate guilt, often about a minor incident, with thoughts of deserved punishment; and, feelings of uselessness or worthlessness as a person. There may be a repudiation of past accomplishments with resultant feelings of failure which are quite incongruent with the patient's actual life history. In its more severe forms, loss of self-esteem may be linked to despair for the future and suicidal ideation. Therefore, the assessment of depression is quite incomplete without a clear appreciation of the patient's self-evaluation.

The opening questions should not suggest any impairment in order to avoid leading the patient's response. *How do you feel about yourself as a person? How do you compare yourself to others?* Subsequent questions should probe specific feelings. *Have you been feeling confident in what you do? Do you have a good opinion of yourself? Have you done anything in particular for which you feel quite guilty? How do you feel about your accomplishments in life so far?* The frequency, duration, and severity of any identified feelings should be clarified. *When you are most down on yourself, do you ever feel useless or worthless as a person?*

Decreased Future Orientation

A depressed mood may have a profound effect upon perception and thought content, including a distorted view of the self, the past, the present, and/or the future. In the midst of depression, it may be very difficult to anticipate any improvement in the mental status or quality of life. Thus, the view of the future may range from pessimism to complete hopelessness. (This is reflected in the colloquial expressions that there is no light at the end of the tunnel or the future is black.) This distorted perception may be enhanced by the cumulative losses experienced by many in the geriatric population which may in turn lead to a realistic appraisal that the future holds very little. Even if effective treatment is offered, the patient may see no point in getting better if it is believed, for example, that all important relationships have been damaged or lost or that the future is bleak even in the absence of depression. Alternatively, severe guilt and remorse for the past may lead one to believe that life in the future is untenable. In some patients, there may be an associated feeling of helplessness to do anything to alter their circumstances such that the future is lost by default. A clinically important index of the severity of depression is the extent to which the patient's future orientation has been decreased. At its extreme—a sense of abject despair or hopelessness—the risk of suicide may be increased.

Inquiry about the patient's view of the future should begin with a direct but open question. *How does the future look to you?* Further questions should probe for specific thought content. *Do you look forward to feeling better? Do you think some form of treatment (or the treatment you are getting) will help you feel better? When you are feeling most depressed or down, do you ever think your future is hopeless? Are you able to do anything to improve your future circumstances?*

Mood-congruent Delusions

The thought content of some patients with very severe depression may be distorted to the point of being delusional. (A delusion is a false belief, which is not commonly held or determined by others of the patient's culture, and which is firmly held by the patient in the presence of logical argument or evidence to the contrary.) In general, the themes of delusional thinking are congruent with the symptoms of depression and are simply the most severe distortions of self-esteem and future orientation (i.e. guilt and deserved severe punishment for non-existent or trivial indiscretions which are believed to be sinful or criminal; the presence of a fatal disease; financial ruin; nihilistic beliefs that past accomplishments, the self or parts of the body, and/or the future and the world do not exist or will be destroyed).

Usually such thought content is quite distressing to the patient and is verbalized during the course of the interview or during the assessment of self-esteem and future orientation. (Generally it should be assessed fully when it is alluded to by the patient in order to preserve the continuity of the interview.) If not, some general probing questions should be used. *Have you been getting any thoughts or ideas which worry or distress you? Do they bother or upset other people when you talk about them? Do you think anything is wrong with your body or your mind? Do you have any strong feelings or beliefs that other people don't seem to share?* Specific questions should then be used to clarify the content of the delusion. In order to confirm that any false beliefs are delusional, rational arguments or evidence against the belief should be presented to the patient to determine whether alternative explanations will be entertained or if the belief is fixed.

Suicidal Ideation: Suicide Risk

The suicide rate peaks in the geriatric age range. Other demographic correlates with suicide that are of particular relevance to the elderly include social isolation (i.e. never married, separated, divorced, widowed; absence of children or other significant relationships; living alone), concurrent alcoholism, and chronic physical illness with resultant disability. A family history of suicide, a history of attempted suicide, and the presence of a mental disorder, particularly depression, are also correlated with an increased risk of suicide. Among the symptoms of depression usually associated with thoughts of suicide are a pervasive and severely depressed mood with anhedonia, a feeling of self-worthlessness, and hopelessness for the future. Therefore, the examination for these symptoms may provide the access to suicidal ideation. The clinical assessment must include an appraisal of the suicide risk. If questions are phrased tactfully and placed in the context of the aforementioned symptoms, they are not offensive and they do not suggest a course of action to the patient. Rather, frank discussion may be therapeutic in that it may be of some relief to the patient to know that the extent of suffering is appreciated by someone who is trying to offer assistance.

Some patients may be quite reluctant to discuss suicidal ideation or to reveal the extent to which they have considered or planned the means of suicide. There may be strong cultural or religious sanctions against suicide so that the patient may feel very guilty or embarrassed. An abrupt question, out of context, about suicide may inhibit a more open discussion and a more accurate appraisal of the suicide risk. Therefore, the line of inquiry about suicide should be a natural extension of the assessment of the mood, self-esteem, and future orientation. As a guideline, it should consist of a series of questions escalating along the continuum of severity of suicidal ideation and behavior.

The initial question should be used to assess whether or not the patient's symptoms have lead to a diminished value of life itself. *When you have been feeling that way—most depressed or down, worthless, hopeless—has life lost any of its value to you? Have you wondered whether or not life was worthwhile?* This can be followed by inquiry about the wish to be dead. *Have you wished you weren't living or hoped you wouldn't wake up from sleep one day?* This passive, morbid ideation is very common and, unto itself, is not indicative of a significant risk of suicide.

The next questions more directly address thoughts of suicide. *Have you thought of doing something that might harm yourself or bring about your death? Have you had any sudden impulses to do something that could have harmed yourself, for example, when driving your car? When you think about it, have you been taking some risks that might have been dangerous for you? When most depressed, have you ever thought of taking your own life?*

An affirmative response to any of these questions leads to detailed inquiry about the thought content, its history (i.e. frequency, duration, intensity, course), and the extent to which the method has been considered or planned. *Have you thought about how you would take your life? Have you made any plans? Have you been putting your affairs in order?* The availability of the means of suicide and its lethality should also be assessed.

Any recent or past history of attempted suicide should be obtained and the lethality of the patient's intent should be assessed. *Have you ever done anything to harm yourself or to attempt to take your life? Could you describe what you did? How were you found? How close were you to killing yourself? What treatment did you receive? Looking back, did you really want to die?* Each suicide attempt should be assessed in full.

In assessing suicide risk, it is also important to determine why the patient has not acted upon thoughts of suicide or why more serious attempts have not been made. In the presence of severe depression, with or without disabling or terminal physical disease and/or desperate social circumstances, most patients retain the will to live. In this regard, it is important to assess the strength of the patient's attachment to relationships, no matter how unsupportive or even destructive they may appear. *What has given you the strength to keep living?* (Often religious or cultural sanctions against suicide or lack of courage are cited in response.) *Do you consider the effect of your death on others?* In this context, it is useful to confirm the presence or absence of any future orientation. *Do you ever think your life (i.e. depression, other illnesses, social/ economic circumstances) will get any better?*

Other Symptoms of Depression

The other symptoms of depression noted in Table 9.2 should also be assessed through observation and direct inquiry. Some examples of specific questions that may be used are presented. *Are you able to think clearly and concentrate on what you are doing? How long can you watch a television show or read?* (It may be easier for the patient to describe a symptom using common behavioral indexes.) *Are you having any difficulty making decisions? Do you have enough energy to do what you want to do? Can you describe any recent change in your appetite or weight?*

Along with the loss of interest or pleasure in other activities, sexual drive may be decreased. This may be assessed independently or while taking the marital history. *How is your physical relationship with your spouse? Have you lost interest in sex?* Since growing old is not synonymous with losing the sex drive, its complete absence may be a significant symptom of depression.

As described in Chapter 4, the symptoms of depression may be masked in the elderly by multiple, and often chronic, somatic complaints. While affective symptoms may be denied, the impact of the somatic symptoms on a patient's mood should be assessed. This may at least facilitate the patient acknowledging the possibility of a connection between the physical and emotional state which may in turn permit the application of "psychological" remedies. *Has experiencing that pain for so long started to get you down? Do you ever notice that the pain is better or worse depending upon your mood?*

(Factors to be considered in the assessment of insomnia are presented in Chapter 11. Paranoid symptoms are described fully in Chapter 7.)

THE EXAMINATION FOR DEMENTIA

The clinical syndrome of dementia has been described in Chapter 5. The natural history of the syndrome is one of progressive loss of nerve cells in the brain. The distribution of that cell loss is extremely variable among regions of the brain subserving specific cognitive functions. Only when the concentration of cell loss in a region reaches a certain level will there be a deficit that can be detected on examination. As a result, there is a great deal of individual variation in the specific cognitive impairments that may be present at any given stage of the illness. The examination for dementia involves testing the major cognitive functions subserved by those areas of the brain in which substantial neuronal loss may occur.

The principal symptoms which may develop during the course of a dementia are summarized in Table 9.3. Guidelines for the clinical assessment of some of the specific symptoms are presented in the ensuing sections. (The cerebral localization of some of these cognitive functions is described in Chapter 5. See Figure 5.2.)

TABLE 9.3
The Symptoms of Dementia

1. Memory loss: initially for recent events
2. Disorientation: time, place, person
3. Decreased concentration
4. Aphasia: impaired reception and expression of language
5. Apraxia: impaired motor integration
6. Impaired abstract thinking
7. Impaired social judgment
8. Lack of insight
9. Personality change: paranoid symptoms
10. Concurrent delirium (See Chapter 6.)

It must be remembered that mental depression may substantially impair performance on tests of cognitive function, so much so that dementia may be diagnosed mistakenly. (The differential diagnosis of depression from dementia may be very difficult and requires a complete assessment of the symptoms of each disorder. The clinical features which best differentiate the two syndromes are described in detail in Chapter 4.) Performance may also be impaired by a lack of motivation and decreased attention. These factors must be considered in assessing the clinical significance of the patient's performance.

Testing cognitive function should not be done hastily as an afterthought at the end of a long interview. Geriatric patients often require considerable time to complete the tests and they may require support and encouragement to persevere. This is particularly the case when cognitive impairment has begun to develop and the patient's capacity for frustration and failure may be declining. (Most of the formal neuropsychological tests involve time limits which have been standardized for young adults. Therefore, normal standards of performance for the elderly may not be well established.)

Early in the course of dementia, patients are usually quite aware of their failing intellect. Naturally, there is a tendency to hide this as much as possible, such that one may encounter considerable reluctance to perform cognitive tests. (The patient may dismiss the tests lightly or become irritable with the examiner.) The patient's reluctance should be acknowledged but s/he should be encouraged to do as well as possible since the objective is to clarify any problems already being experienced. In the presence of more severe cognitive impairment, the patient's anxiety may increase markedly as repeated attempts to perform a task are unsuccessful. This may reach the point of an inappropriately strong emotional response such as extreme anger or a sudden outburst of crying with an attempt to leave the room. This is referred to as a catastrophic reaction. (The stress of testing should not be avoided just to prevent such a reaction but appropriate support should be given if it occurs. In this regard, the time and setting of the interview and the attention paid to establishing rapport with the patient are important.)

The assessment of cognitive functioning may be introduced to the patient with a very general question or statement. *Have you noticed any difficulty with your memory or concentration lately? I would now like to ask a few questions to see if you are having any trouble with your memory or concentration.*

Since dementing patients may respond to questions with dismissive or superficially correct statements, an attempt must be made to obtain explicit responses to specific questions. It is preferable to document the patient's actual response since the interpretation of errors on specific tests may be quite difficult as noted in the ensuing sections. (In this regard, many screening tests of cognitive function include a numerical scoring system which may or may not be linked to specific descriptions of the possible abnormal responses. Furthermore, the total score may be influenced unduly by a disproportionate weighting of the tests of one or more specific functions. Therefore, in using such screening instruments, it is preferable to record and summarize the patient's responses to each test.) Initial screening questions or tests are usually quite simple and are intended to detect quite gross impairments. As such, they may be of limited usefulnes in the assessment of patients early in the course of dementia. Similarly, they may not detect substantive impairment in those patients whose premorbid level of functioning in specific areas was very high. Therefore, more difficult questions or tests may be necessary to probe those areas in which impairment has been suggested by the history. (Referral for standardized neuropsychological testing may be required.)

Disorientation

Varying degrees of disorientation occur during the course of dementia, usually secondary to memory loss but sometimes due to concurrent delirium. When disorientation is severe, the lack of awareness of or attention to the immediate environment may preclude much of the cognitive assessment. Therefore, it is useful to examine orientation at the beginning of the assessment. The level of consciousness observed during the assessment interview should be noted. Similarly, the patient's ability to pay attention during the interview should be described (i.e. distractibility, difficulty shifting from one question to the next). The objective is then to determine the patient's ability to give a good account of the time, his/her whereabouts, the people in the immediate environment, and the purpose of the interview.

Orientation to time may be assessed with a few specific questions. *What is today's date (day, month, year)? What day of the week is it? Without looking at your watch, approximately what time of day is it?* Supplemental questions may be necessary to assess the full degree of disorientation. *How long have you lived here? What season of the year is it?* (If applicable) *What important event or holiday occurred recently?* It must be remembered that institutionalized or house-bound patients may have little need or motivation to note the passage of time. Therefore, minor errors are common and their significance must be interpreted within the context of the results of the overall examination and the circumstances.

Orientation to place may also be assessed with a series of specific questions. *What is the full address of this house/apartment/building (apartment and street number, street name, city, province)? What is the name of this place? What type of place is it (i.e. apartment building, nursing home, hospital)?* Further questions should be asked when significant errors occur and/or to assess the patient's orientation to the contiguous environment. This is particularly important if there is a history of the patient wandering away from home and/or getting lost. *What is the nearest major street intersection and how would you get there? How do you get to the grocery store from here?* (Other questions should be related to any history of disorientation under specific circumstances.) Minor errors in orientation to place are common and usually insignificant when made by patients who have moved recently.

Orientation to person is usually impaired only when dementia is quite advanced and when other deficits are prominent. It is usually indicated by a history of misidentifying people, often close relatives. (In this regard, it may be the harbinger of a delusional belief that a close relative has been replaced by a double.) A few specific questions should be asked. *Do you recall who I (the examiner) am? What is my job and why am I here? Can you tell me who is this person (pointing to any relative in attendance or to a photograph in the room)?*

Memory Loss

The greatest concentration of neuronal loss in primary degenerative dementia or Alzheimer's disease occurs in that area of the brain which is required to commit new learning or experiences into memory. Therefore, all patients present with impaired recent memory, usually early during their course of illness. Remote memory becomes impaired later in the course. Memory function involves the processes of registration, retention and retrieval (recall and recognition) of information. The clinical assessment of recent memory is illustrated in Figure 9.1. This method of assessment is based upon the model of memory processing which was described in Chapter 5. There are innumerable screening tests of memory but only one suggested method will be described.

FIGURE 9.1

The Clinical Assessment of Recent Memory

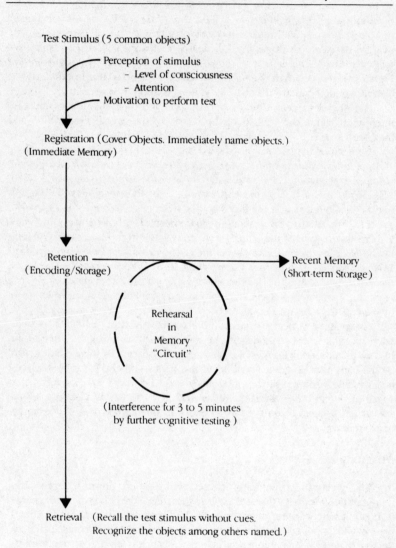

Test Stimulus (5 common objects)

— Perception of stimulus
- Level of consciousness
- Attention
— Motivation to perform test

Registration (Cover Objects. Immediately name objects.)
(Immediate Memory)

Retention ———————————————————→ Recent Memory
(Encoding/Storage)   (Short-term Storage)

Rehearsal
in
Memory
"Circuit"

(Interference for 3 to 5 minutes
by further cognitive testing)

Retrieval   (Recall the test stimulus without cues.
Recognize the objects among others named.)

The first stage in committing the test stimulus or new information to memory storage involves its registration. The registration of information, also referred to as immediate memory, does not last more than a few seconds after the information is presented. Since memory storage per se is not involved, this process is not impaired in dementia. However, it may be disrupted by anything which reduces consciousness, attention, or motivation to perform the test, including delirium and depression. Registration may be assessed most conveniently with the information to be used in the test of retention.

Any five unrelated common objects (i.e. key, coin, cotton ball, pen, comb) should be held in the examiner's hand and shown to the patient who should be asked to name and remember the objects. The objects are then covered and the patient should be asked immediately to name them. (If necessary, up to three trials are given for this test of registration. If the patient is unsuccessful, *three* new objects should be presented and the test repeated.) The patient should then be told to remember the objects because s/he will be asked to name them again after a few minutes. It must be emphasized that both the test of registration and the explicit instructions to ensure awareness of the test expectation are prerequisites for the subsequent assessment of retention and retrieval. (Many tests of memory use only three items of information. In practice with the elderly, this task is usually too simple such that five objects are suggested for initial screening purposes.)

Recent memory (short-term retention or storage) is assessed by asking the patient to recall (retrieve from storage) the test stimulus after approximately three to five minutes. During this interval, conscious rehearsal of the stimulus is minimized by keeping the objects out of sight and by interfering with rehearsal through presentation of competing information to which the patient must attend. (This should be done simply by continuing the cognitive assessment through the five-minute test interval.) It must be noted that the immediate recall of any test stimulus, for example a series of digits, without the previously noted interval is not a test of recent memory since no retention or storage capacity is required.

The initial request to retrieve the information should be phrased so as to avoid any suggestion of the correct answer. *Can you recall what I asked you to remember?* The response may range from a complete lack of awareness of the test to recitation of the five objects in the sequence in which they were arranged. If the former occurs, a succession of cues should be given to gauge the severity of the memory loss. An open palm can be extended with repetition of the initial request. The request can be rephrased. *Can you recall what was in my hand a few minutes ago? Can you remember the things that were in my hand?* If less than five objects are recalled, further cues should be provided. *There were five objects. Do you remember the rest of them?* When the limit of free recall has been reached, several objects should be named, including the missing test objects. Retrieval by recognition may occur when the patient is asked to identify the correct objects from among those named. The patient's responses at each successive prompt should be recorded. Patients without dementia are usually able to recall four or five objects without much prompting.

Remote memory (long-term retention or storage) is assessed during the course of the interview when the patient is asked to provide historical information. Loss of memory for relatively unimportant details of events (i.e. children's ages, ages of parents' deaths) is a common accompaniment of normal ageing. Loss of memory for important events (i.e. number of children, birthdate) is clinically significant.

Decreased Concentration

The capacity to sustain concentration through a sequence of mental operations is often impaired during the course of dementia. The original objective of the task may be forgotten such that repeated redirection is required. Alternatively, the patient may be unable to shift easily from element to element of the sequence so that the same error may be repeated throughout. Concentration should be assessed by having the patient perform an arithmetic or verbal task which requires a sequence of responses. *Subtract 7 from 100 and continue to subtract 7 from your answer until you reach 0. Name the months of the year backwards, starting with December.*

Aphasia

Impairment of the ability to understand or express language may be a prominent symptom of dementia. (Impaired hearing as a possible cause must be excluded.) When present it may affect the performance on other tests of cognitive function since the patient may not be able to comprehend instructions or express answers. Therefore, screening tests for dementia should include those for receptive and expressive aphasia.

The ability to understand speech is assessed during the course of the interview as the patient responds to questions. Impairment may be evidenced by apparently irrelevant responses. It may be formally tested by asking the patient to follow a complex verbal command. *Pick up this paper, fold it in half, and place it on the floor.* (A similar command should be presented in writing to assess the ability to comprehend written language.)

The expression of speech should also be noted during the interview. Progressive dementia may be characterized by difficulty finding the right word, inability to name objects (nominal aphasia), incorrect word substitutions (paraphasia, including new words), loss of specific parts of speech (nouns, verbs, conjunctions), decreased fluency, and unintelligible speech. The ability to correctly name objects is impaired in almost all patients with expressive aphasia. Therefore, screening of this function should be included in the assessment. Initial screening is undertaken during the assessment of memory when the patient is asked to name objects to be remembered. Later, the examiner should point to objects in the room asking the patient to name each (i.e. ceiling, floor, telephone, watch, shirt, shoe). The sensitivity of the test to early impairment should be increased by asking the patient to identify parts of objects since the words are less commonly used (i.e. floor tile, telephone receiver, watch crystal, shirt collar). Patients with nominal aphasia may identify one or more of the objects by an incorrect name, by explaining the function of the object verbally or with hand gestures, or by giving related information. For example, a watch may be identified as "You use it to tell the time." or a telephone as "I have a green box at home and its number is (the patient's correct telephone number)." Interestingly, the inability to name the same objects may not occur during more spontaneous conversation. For example, the same patient may use the word "telephone" appropriately during the interview.

The loss of conjunctions may develop early in the course of expressive aphasia. Therefore, the patient should be asked to repeat the following phrase: "No *if*'s, *and*'s, or *but*'s."

The patient should be asked to write a sentence without specifying the content. This is a very complex task requiring the integration of language and motor function. Some patients may require considerable prompting, even to the point of the examiner dictating a short sentence. The amount of prompting required should be noted. Some patients write their name since the signature may be well preserved despite gross impairment in writing. They should be asked to try to write any other words.

Apraxia and Impaired Constructional Ability

Various complex motor functions may be impaired during the course of dementia. Some of these functions require the integration of extensive areas of the cerebral cortex so that they are vulnerable to disruption early in the course of dementia. Therefore, the assessment of motor integration is an integral part of the examination for dementia.

Apraxia is the inability to perform previously learned complex motor tasks. Patients with ideomotor apraxia cannot demonstrate tasks on verbal command. The approximate movements must be mimicked without any non-verbal cues. *Show me how to use a toothbrush. Show me how to flip a coin.* If the patient is unable to mimic the action, s/he can usually imitate the examiner or demonstrate using the real object.

Patients with ideational apraxia are unable to integrate a series of steps in order to perform a complex task (i.e. fold a letter, place it in an envelope, seal it, and place a stamp on the envelope). Almost all patients with this form of apraxia have impaired auditory comprehension, constructional impairment and/or visual-spatial disorientation.

Dressing apraxia results from the inability to orientate clothing to the appropriate body part. For example, the patient may repeatedly insert the right arm into the left sleeve and then try to rotate the shirt around the body.

Constructional ability requires the complex integration of visual-spatial and motor functions involving the occipital, parietal and frontal lobes. Because of the extensive cortical area necessary to perform constructional tasks, this function is frequently impaired by diffuse cortical disease. Therefore, tests of this function are most likely to detect neuronal degeneration in the cortex quite early in the course of dementia.

Constructional ability should be assessed initially by asking the patient to reproduce a standard geometric design. The design should be on plain white paper. The patient should be given a pencil and instructed to copy the design on the same page. *Please draw this design exactly as it looks to you.* This two-dimensional line drawing task can be supplemented with three-dimensional tasks which require the patient to copy designs using a set of blocks or match sticks. (Since the design to be copied remains in view, these constructional tasks do not require an intact memory.) The patient should also be asked to draw a common object from memory. As opposed to the aforementioned tasks, this requires the patient to invoke a mental image of the object. A clock face is suggested so that an intact recent memory is not required. *Please draw the face of a clock; draw the hands to show the time as 10 past 11.*

Both the manner in which the patient performs the tasks and the final results should be observed. The signs of impaired constructional ability may be summarized as follows:

1. Difficulty with overall orientation. Repeated rotation of the paper before starting to draw. Uncertainty about where to place the drawing on the page. Crowding the drawing into a corner of the page or overlapping the test design. Difficulty initiating the drawing with frequent approaches to the paper with the pencil.
2. Repetition of part of the drawing or placement of one block. The same line or angle may be traced over and over, creating a dog-eared appearance. The same block may be rotated and replaced several times. (This is an example of perseveration; the patient is unable to shift attention easily from one part of the stimulus to another.)
3. Gross distortion of the figure, usually due to incorrect angles or dislocation of individual elements. (Often clock hands are pointed to 10 and 11 instead of the more "abstract" 11 and 2.)
4. Complete separation of elements of the design or omission of parts of the figure.
5. Trial and error with little apparent learning from each successive attempt so that the same incorrect construction is repeated.
6. Satisfaction with a grossly incorrect construction. Inability to point out the errors.

Examples of patients' dyspraxic drawings of a geometric design and a clock face are presented in Figure 9.2.

Other Symptoms of Dementia

The highest integrative or intellectual functions of the cerebral cortex are very vulnerable to diffuse cortical disease. In general terms, they may be grouped as follows: abstract thinking and reasoning, including the manipulation of knowledge to solve problems; and, social judgment. The ability to perform effectively and/or safely in the community is, in large part, determined by the capacity of these complex intellectual functions. Therefore, they should be assessed during the examination for signs and symptoms of dementia. In most instances, the patient or informant will complain of impairment in these functions, particularly that of social judgment (i.e. inappropriate reduction of sexual,

FIGURE 9.2
Examples of Impaired Constructional Ability

Test Design   **Copies by Patients**

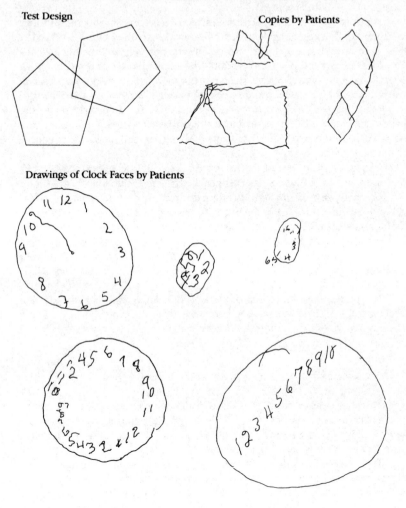

Drawings of Clock Faces by Patients

financial, or other social inhibitions). Ancillary questioning can be used to substantiate the complaints.

Abstract thinking should be assessed by requiring the patient to explain the similarity between pairs of overtly different objects. Explicit instructions should be given. *I am going to name some pairs of objects which are similar or like each other in some way. Please tell me how they are similar. Apple–Orange. Desk—Bookcase. Poem—Painting. Horse—Apple.* Abstract responses are fruit, furniture, works of art, and living things. Impaired abstraction is indicated by description of the specific properties of the items, differences between the items, and generalizations without reference to the items. (It should be noted that performance on this test may be largely dependent upon the patient's education and/or global premorbid intelligence. Interpretation of the responses must be made in that context.)

The application of knowledge to solve problems and social judgment may be assessed by presenting hypothetical situations to the patient and asking how s/he would respond. To provide information relevant to the patient's functional capacity, the situations should be applicable to daily living. *What would you do if your furnace stopped working during a very cold weekend in the winter? How would you go about planning a trip to visit your relative/ birthplace/specific city or country?* Any number of situations relevant to the patient may be used. (The assessment of financial competence and safety may be aided by this line of inquiry.) A judgment should be made about the adequacy of the patient's responses.

Insight, or awareness of the presence of specific disabilities, may be lost during the course of dementia. This may be assessed with specific questions. *Do you think there is anything wrong with your memory or ability to think? Are you having any difficulty looking after yourself or doing your job?* (Specific dysfunctions obtained during the history should be mentioned.) Incongruities between the patient's responses and actual circumstances should be probed. *Can you tell me the reasons for your early retirement? Can you tell me your reasons for moving to this nursing home? Why have I been asked to talk to you today?*

The protean manifestations of personality change and paranoid ideation which may occur in dementia have been described in Chapters 5 and 7. These features are assessed during the history taking. Similarly, the symptoms of concurrent delirium are presented in Chapter 6.

CONCLUSION

The clinical assessment of geriatric patients who present with symptoms of mental disorders is often very difficult and time-consuming. Appropriate interviewing techniques must be used and adapted as necessary to elicit information which is often quite inaccessible.

The objective of an assessment is to reach an accurate diagnosis upon which to base specific treatment and case management plans. Diagnostic accuracy is largely dependent upon an appreciation of the full constellation of symptoms and behavior with which the patient presents. Thus, accurate observations from many sources may be required for a complete examination.

The examiner should be knowledgeable about the many symptoms which constitute those mental disorders or syndromes which occur most commonly in the elderly. The decision that a patient meets the diagnostic criteria for any given disorder should be based on an adequate assessment of all its constituent symptoms. It must be remembered that many symptoms and behaviors are common to a number of mental disorders such that incomplete examination greatly increases the probability of diagnostic error. That may be a gross disservice to the patient if it leads to a misleading prognosis and inappropriate management.

REFERENCES AND SUGGESTED READINGS

American Psychiatric Association. 1980. *Diagnostic and Statistical Manual of Mental Disorders*. 3rd ed. American Psychiatric Association.

Anthony K., L. Le Resche and U. Niaz et al. 1982. "Limits of the 'Mini-Mental State' as a Screening Test for Dementia and Delirium among Hospital Patients." *Psychological Medicine*. 12: 397.

Capwell R. R., N. B. Lee and D. Robertson. 1982. "The Clinical History and Physical Examination in the Older Patient." *Modern Medicine*. 37: 195.

Critchley M. 1969. *The Parietal Lobes*. New York: Hafner Publishing Co.

Folstein M. F., S. E. Folstein and P. R. McHugh. 1975. "'Mini-Mental State'. A Practical Method for Grading the Cognitive State of Patients for the Clinician." *Journal of Psychiatric Research*. 12: 189.

Geschwind N. 1970. "The Organization of Language and the Brain." *Science*. 170: 940.

Geschwind N. 1971. "Current Concepts: Aphasia." *New England Journal of Medicine*. 284: 654.

Martin B. A., A. M. Peter and M. R. Eastwood. 1983. "The Mental Status Examination for Dementia: A Review of Practice in a Psychiatric Hospital." *Canadian Journal of Psychiatry*. 28: 287.

Shulman K. I., R. Shedletsky and I. L. Silver. 1986. "The Challenge of Time: Clock-drawing and Cognitive Function in the Elderly." *International Journal of Geriatric Psychiatry*. In press.

Spitzer R. L., B. W. Williams and A. E. Skodol. 1980. "DSM-III: The Major Achievements and An Overview." *American Journal of Psychiatry*. 137: 151.

Strub R. L. and F. W. Black. 1977. *The Mental Status Examination in Neurology*. Philadelphia: E. A. Davis.

Wells C. E. (ed.) 1977. *Dementia*. 2nd ed. Philadelphia: F. A. Davis.

Wells C. E. 1979. "Pseudodementia." *American Journal of Psychiatry*. 136: 895.

10

Management of Difficult Behavior

E. Anne Lennox, R.N., B.Sc.N., M.P.H. and
Deborah M. Clark, B.S.W., C.S.W., M.Ed.

This chapter will address specific behavioral problems which challenge families and professional caregivers who are committed to maintaining the mentally impaired in the community. These behavioral problems may occur in the course of many specific mental disorders described earlier in this book (for example, depression, dementia, and paranoid disorders). The overall objective of community-based care is only appropriate when a reasonable quality of life and degree of dignity can be preserved for both elderly relative and caregiver. In certain situations, behavior problems secondary to mental disorders may lead to unacceptable physical risk. There may be social consequences of diminished judgment which are not life threatening but may fail to meet acceptable social standards. Premature or inappropriate placement may be perceived as the only alternative when the emotional and physical burden overwhelms the caregiver. Effective management of behavior problems may mitigate the stress to caregivers, and increase the likelihood of continued community care. Management of the following behaviors will be considered: sleep disturbances and sundowning, wandering, sexual disinhibition, incontinence, paranoid behavior, and hostility and aggression. The example of driving as a safety issue will also be presented. A brief section addressing communication with the mentally impaired elderly has been included.

SOCIAL FACTORS

There are social factors which will either increase or decrease the probability of achieving the objective of community care for the elderly. For example, care of the mentally impaired older person becomes more problematic in the absence of a competent caregiver. A professional helper's assessment and intervention must reflect an understanding of the unique social factors in the caregiving situation. Social factors will be considered, with a focus on the impact to the caregiving situation. The following factors will be discussed: mental status, family support, self care, safety, and personality attributes.

When the elderly person is mentally impaired and living in an unsafe situation by community standards, it may be difficult for caregivers to advocate for the right to self-determination and privacy. If there is uncertainty about an individual's mental competence, a psychogeriatric assessment by a qualified health professional is strongly recommended. Part of this assessment process includes a review of the individual's medical history and current physical status. Acute or chronic physical illnesses which cannot be adequately controlled in the home may accelerate the need for institutionalization.

The importance of the family in maintaining the older individual in the community has been emphasized in Chapter 14. An assessment of the family relationships and resources is required in order to determine the type and frequency of assistance the family is willing to provide. For example, if a family were previously uninvolved and detached, it is unlikely that their help can be enlisted to provide support in times of need. The fact that many families are geographically separated makes it difficult for a daughter in Calgary to co-ordinate her mother's care in Toronto. If the family is unavailable to assist, it is important to assess the older individual's informal support system. Long-time friends, neighbors, or good-hearted landlords may offer help, provided there is professional consultation.

An older person's ability to remain at home safely is contingent upon the capacity to perform activities of daily living either independently or with appropriate support. If on assessment, some degree of impairment is found, can assistive devices or training be provided to offset the disability? When the degree of impairment is beyond self-management, can community support services such as Meals-on-Wheels or Homemaking be involved to compensate for functional deficits? A further consideration will be the individual's and/or family's willingness to accept outside support. Involving the older person, particularly the mentally competent individual in the decision-making process is a fundamental principle in care of the elderly.

Safety issues are an extremely important aspect of community-based care. Areas to be considered cluster around unsafe behaviors such as smoking, driving, wandering, non-compliance with medication, or environmental hazards such as poor shelter. If the individual has a problem in one or more of these areas, the feasibility of care at home is decreased. However, there will always be older individuals who will choose to remain at home despite significant threats to health and safety.

Consideration of the older individual's personality factors, including coping style, is a necessary part of formulating the decision as to the most appropriate location for care. Lifelong personality traits such as stubbornness, stoicism, or a domineering character may preclude the elder's acceptance of support from informal and formal sources, thereby complicating the advocate's commitment to quality community-based care. There is no formula for establishing exactly when and where a person should be institutionalized; the decision should always be based upon situation-specific information. To summarize, there are factors which influence the decision regarding the location of care. These can be grouped into three main categories; those associated with the individual, such as personality, mental competence, physical health and functional abilities; those associated with the support system, i.e. family and community resources; and safety and environmental issues.

SLEEP DISTURBANCES AND SUNDOWNING

Family caregivers may be further stressed by sleep disturbances of the elderly relative. These sleep disturbances may take the form of nighttime wakefulness with increased agitation. When an elderly person experiences an increase in behavioral problems and confusion in the early evening, it is referred to as sundowning. Caregivers may become exhausted as a result of this disruptive behavior, thus limiting their abilities to cope on a long-term basis.

Common sense approaches to sleep disturbances are limiting daytime napping and increasing the impaired person's physical activity and stimulation. Another useful strategy to reduce nighttime agitation is to plan the individual's day so that fewer demands and expectations are made in the evening hours.

If a person's nighttime agitation is consistently disruptive to the household, low dose neuroleptics such as Haldol or Loxapine are drugs of choice. Traditional hypnotics and sedatives are of limited value and may lead to unwanted side effects such as increased agitation and confusion in vulnerable individuals. These drugs may be effective during an acute episode of nighttime agitation, but lose their efficacy with long-term administration. If the individual's sleep disturbance is a symptom of a major depression it may be worthwhile to use a more sedating anti-depressant such as Sinequan. If medications are used, periodic review to assess effectiveness and to observe for the presence of side effects is the recommended management approach. (Refer to Chapter 11 for a more detailed review of psychotropic medications.)

WANDERING

One of the associated behaviors in progressive dementias may be wandering, which is a serious problem for lay and professional caregivers. A person with a history of wandering will frequently be denied admission to a day care program. The admission policy of many long-term care facilities may exclude wanderers because institutions are not designed structurally to protect a person from leaving the premises. Concern about legal liability and safety issues prevail. Wandering as a behavioral problem makes care of the impaired person at home or in an institution a very stressful undertaking for caregivers.

Wandering refers to walking that occurs independent of normal environmental cues. Several patterns of wandering will be described. For example, what may have started as purposeful behavior may evolve into a wandering episode as the disoriented individual seeks to find his/her way. For others, wandering may be caused by disorientation and confusion resulting from nocturnal agitation. Another form may be the result of agitated pacing. A particularly troublesome pattern of wandering is characterized by determined efforts to exit. Wandering may also occur in situations where new learning is required which exceeds the person's capacity to adjust. It may be aimless, occurring for no specific reason. A functional analysis of an individual's wandering is essential before implementing a management strategy. For example, the person who has a single episode will not pose the same management problem as the persistent and determined wanderer. As can be seen, the term is used to refer to a variety of different behavioral patterns associated with ambulation.

Wandering behavior fulfils a unique purpose for the individual. The health professional's recognition of its significance and possible precipitants will facilitate effective management. Reality orientation as a treatment for wandering should be used selectively as it may result in increased anxiety and frustration, precipitating more frequent wandering episodes. For example, a concrete interpretation of reality orientation would direct the caregiver to confront the wanderer seeking a parent with the fact that mother died thirty years ago and the family home is no longer in existence. An alternate approach would be to validate the wanderer's underlying longing for security and comfort. The use of reminiscence and family memorabilia is more humane and less threatening to the mentally impaired person. The professional's effective utilization of tactful distraction may yield more positive results with the wanderer than direct verbal confrontation or physical and/or chemical restraint. Caregivers should utilize strategies that will help them explore the wandering agenda of the impaired person (for example, wandering may be expression of boredom, restlessness, or increased anxiety).

In addition to the above strategies, several practical recommendations are offered:

1. Obtain a medic-alert bracelet for identification.
2. Notify local police and provide a photograph of the wanderer.
3. Notify neighbors, letter carriers, and people in the surrounding area of the problem.
4. Install new locks (the person may be unable to learn how to use a new lock no matter how simple): place them lower down on the door, closer to the floor.
5. Increase daily physical activity.
6. Supervision should be proportional to safety risk.
7. Install an alarm system.

In institutions, the following suggestions are recommended:

1. Establish a search protocol for the institution. All staff should be aware of residents who wander.
2. Document the fact on the medical chart that a person is a wanderer.
3. Provide sufficient space within the institution for physical exercise.
4. Promote outdoor activity for the person who wanders.
5. Pay attention to hazardous areas within the institution.

SEXUAL DISINHIBITION

The occurrence of sexually inappropriate behavior in an older person for the first time is often related to diminished judgment and disinhibition. An older person's interest in sexual relations is not of itself inappropriate; however, it is the *when* and *where* that create problems. Sexually inappropriate behavior may include exhibitionism, masturbation in public areas, or fondling. Inappropriate sexual behavior may be seen in several conditions, that is, drug induced delirium, post-stroke, or associated with a progressive dementia. It is important to do a thorough assessment of the behavior problem in order to take the most appropriate action. Some medications may increase an elderly person's confusion and agitation which could result in an individual acting inappropriately, such as accidentally climbing into another person's bed or exposing him/herself. A periodic review of the individual's medication will help to minimize problems and paradoxical reactions. Some individuals who have had a stroke may display unsuitable sexual behavior for the first time as a result of a loss of inhibiting brain functions. Inappropriate sexual behavior may also be a secondary feature of a dementia as the result of disinhibition (similar to a stroke victim) or disorientation.

Both professional and family caregivers should be informed that brain damage may reduce the demented individual's self-control. Exhibitionism in Alzheimer's disease is often related to forgetfulness in that the individual may not remember where s/he is, how to dress, and the importance of being dressed. If an elderly impaired person engages in masturbation in public areas, this will likely cause upset and distress to staff and/or family members. An effective approach when confronted with this behavior is to remain calm and direct the person to a private place. Abrupt interference or a condescending attitude on the part of the staff or family may antagonize the individual and precipitate further problems. In an institutional setting, limiting access to public areas or changing rooms may help in cases where an individual is making sexual advances towards a less competent individual.

Family caregivers should be encouraged to seek advice from a physician or other health professionals about a relative's disturbing sexual behavior.

INCONTINENCE

Urinary incontinence is a major geriatric problem with medical, psychological, social, and economic implications. Of those 65 years and older, estimates are that 10 to 20 percent in the community, and more than 50 percent of elderly in long-term care facilities suffer some degree of urinary incontinence. No convincing association with gender, increasing age, or urinary infection has ever been reported (Ouslander et al. 1982). As it is one of the most difficult conditions for the elderly and families to manage at home, incontinence frequently leads to institutionalization. Because it is often viewed by elderly people, families, and health professionals as an inevitable consequence of old age, it is frequently left unevaluated and untreated. Emphasis is placed on keeping the person dry and clean, and little is done to treat the underlying cause of the incontinence.

Incontinence is not a disease; it is a non-specific symptom of an underlying medical, psychiatric, or environmental problem. It has multiple physiological causes, among which are neurologic disease, prostatic disease, uterine prolapse, and urinary tract infection. Psychiatric illnesses found in the elderly in conjunction with incontinence are hypomanic or agitated states, dementias, schizophrenia, acute confusional states, or psychotic depression. Environmental factors con- tributing to incontinence include location of the toilet, and the distance to it.

Treatment depends on a full accurate assessment of the problem. Physical examination by a physician to diagnose causes of urinary incontinence would include abdominal, pelvic, rectal, vaginal, and urological assessment. A home assessment would include attention to the following details:

1. When did the problem begin?
2. What are the voiding patterns, both day and night? Are there diurnal variations in frequency?
3. What is the number of voids per day and the number of accidents per day? When do they occur?
4. Quantity of urine—Is there continuous leaking or a large amount of urine passed once or twice during the day?
5. Physical setting—What is the distance to the toilet? Are stairs a barrier?
6. General mobility—Is the person bed bound or is mobility difficult? Does s/he sit all day in a chair that is difficult to get out of?
7. Assess manual dexterity—Is the person able to remove clothing in time?
8. Mental status—Is the person aware of the need to void? Is s/he aware of the incontinence? It is also important to know the person's perception of whether incontinence is a problem. Can the person find the toilet? Does s/he have the mental ability to dress and undress? Does s/he have the ability to carry out a series of behaviors in the toiletting sequence? Are there problems with aphasia, that is, can the person request toiletting when needed?
9. Drugs—Medications can contribute to the loss of control of urine. Examples are diuretics, sedatives, hypnotics, tricyclic antidepressants, anti-Parkinsonian agents, or over-the-counter drugs (decongestants and diet pills).
10. Daily hydration—Try to obtain an input/output record. Is the caregiver unduly restricting fluids to avoid incontinence?
11. General condition—Is there an acute or a chronic illness? For example, uncontrolled diabetes could be a cause of incontinence.
12. Caregiver's reactions to incontinence—What is the family's attitude to the problem?

Incontinence in persons with a dementing illness usually relates to progressive neuronal loss. The person may be unable to plan ahead in order to carry out the toiletting sequence, that is, the individual may realize the urge to void, but forgets where the toilet is or how to get there. Caregivers can be taught timed voiding techniques. The caregiver must take the person to the toilet every one or two hours routinely. Fluid intake must be normal or greater to accomplish this successfully. The goal of timed voiding techniques is to keep the bladder empty through use of this fixed routine. The only criteria is that the person be mobile and co-operative with the primary caregiver.

It should not be assumed that incontinence in the elderly population is irreversible unless a thorough evaluation and comprehensive treatment plan has been conducted. This principle applies equally to the mentally impaired individual.

PARANOID SYMPTOMS

An associated feature of a primary dementia may be paranoid symptoms. Paranoia may range from mild suspiciousness to fixed false beliefs of persecution, jealousy, or influence. Suspicious or paranoid ideas may develop as a result of a distortion or misinterpretation of reality. The person may begin to rely on the defence mechanism of projection, that is, blaming others in order to deny failing memory. This behavior is among the most disturbing symptom in early dementia, particularly to caregivers who may be the object of the fixed ideas of suspected infidelity, theft, or persecution.

Delusions are persistent false beliefs held by an individual that cannot be altered by a rational explanation. In dementia, the delusional beliefs are often less elaborate and poorly systematized. The beliefs may be generalized, or may become more focal with one or a number of themes developing. For example, landlords, neighbors, or people of different racial backgrounds may be the targets in addition to immediate family members. People with a dementing illness may develop unshakable ideas that belongings have been stolen, or that people want to harm them. Individuals may also experience hallucinations, that is, hearing, seeing, feeling, or smelling things that are not there. Such hallucinations may be terrifying for the individual and extremely upsetting for family members because of the association with "insanity". Caregivers need to know whether these symptoms, particularly auditory hallucinations, occur as the result of brain injury, are caused by a superimposed delirium from drugs, or by an acute illness.

For some people, suspiciousness is a lifelong personality style which becomes exaggerated as a result of psychosocial and cognitive changes in later life. Of particular importance is a loss of sensory ability, specifically hearing. Paranoid ideas are a frequent accompaniment of hearing loss. The individual responds to impaired communication by projecting difficulties onto others.

Suggested strategies for community management of suspiciousness and paranoia are as follows:

1. Help the person regain some sense of control over his/her life, by allowing decision-making opportunities where possible.
2. Try to compensate for losses. This may range from the use of a hearing aid to specific help with organizing possessions or the use of memory enhancement techniques.
3. It is important to counsel family members to accept a person's accusations as behavioral symptoms of a disease, rather than a personal assault. This will help reduce hostility and social isolation directed toward the person experiencing the paranoid ideas.
4. Observe if major environmental changes were associated with the development of paranoid thinking. Confusion in a new setting and subsequent anxiety often precipitate increased suspiciousness.

5. Anti-anxiety medication may be helpful when used in conjunction with psychosocial measures such as counselling the family. A trial of a neuroleptic medication such as Haldol or Loxapine in geriatric doses is recommended if the person's emotional or functional ability is significantly impaired by the paranoid ideas. (See also Chapter 7.)

HOSTILITY AND AGGRESSION

Aggressive behavior may be a secondary feature of dementia. Caregivers may seek the advice of professionals when they cannot cope with a relative's aggressive outbursts. It is worth noting that many behavioral problems escalate when the individual has an intercurrent medical illness. Proper management of the medical status is therefore essential.

Behavior disturbances such as hostility and aggression may be amenable to a combination of psychopharmacology, environmental modification, and family education. Before initiating treatment, it is important to obtain a history from the caregiver regarding the frequency, severity, and extent of the problem. If the individual's irritability and aggression are a daily occurrence and significantly interfere with caregiving tasks, then the use of a neuroleptic such as Haldol or Loxapine in geriatric dosages is the treatment of choice. The choice of an anti-psychotic medication should be based on the side effect profile of the drug and the medical status of the individual. With the administration of a neuroleptic, it is important to observe for extrapyramidal side effects. (See Chapter 11.)

Caregivers must be helped to understand that these physical and verbal outbursts are part of the dementing illness. Catastrophic reactions occur when the demented individual is overwhelmed by the expectations of others and responds by emotional overreaction to the situation. These reactions may range from mild annoyance to physically aggressive acts. A caregiver may view the relative's overreaction as obstinate or moody behavior. Educating caregivers to identify precipitants of the reaction while remaining calm and controlled are key strategies. In addition, teaching families to gently divert their relative's attention in these situations may further reduce the frequency and impact of the catastrophic reaction.

DRIVING

Impaired mental functioning may affect an individual's performance of previously well-learned activities. For example, driving may be a well rehearsed skill for an elderly person; however, it requires a complex interaction of eyes, brain, and muscle, and the ability to problem-solve quickly. Co-ordination, reaction time, and mental alertness are essential to safe driving. An individual may make an independent decision to discontinue driving. For others, driving may be associated with a lifelong occupation, independence, or a "macho" image. In these situations elderly individuals may fiercely resist even the mildest suggestion to curtail driving. Sometimes driving behavior is the first marker event to family members of a significant change in the relative's abilities. For example, an elderly relative may lose sense of direction on a familiar route to the extent of becoming disoriented and lost. It is encumbent upon the health professional to enquire about such significant changes in a routine functional assessment. If the assessment reveals a recent history of impaired driving performance, the health professional must document and report this to the family physician. Unfortunately, early signs of mental impairment may go unrecognized and the person continues to drive. Difficulty driving may be part of a cluster of signs indicating impaired cognitive abilities which slowly undermine an elderly person's independence and self-esteem.

The Highway Traffic Act (1980) states that a physician must file a report with the Registrar of the Ministry of Transportation for every person, who in his/her opinion, is suffering from a condition that makes it dangerous to continue driving. There may be a temporary revocation of a driver's licence after an acute illness, requiring a driver's test for renewal. In the case of a progressive mental disorder, suspension of the driver's licence would be permanent.

Removing a person's licence may trigger a catastrophic reaction, or be the precipitant of a depressive episode for someone who is aware of his/her limitations. If the person is unwilling to stop driving, family members can be advised to hide the keys or remove the distributor cap from the car.

COMMUNICATION WITH THE MENTALLY IMPAIRED ELDERLY

Elderly people with behavior problems secondary to a mental disorder may have distinct communication difficulties. Effective management of behavior is contingent upon the recognition of these unique problems of communication. Communication difficulties take the form of expressive and receptive aphasias. Aphasia has been defined as a disturbance of established language ability secondary to altered brain function. This means that the affected individual will have difficulty attaching meaning to incoming messages, and/or organizing the messages to be sent. Guidelines for communicating with the mentally impaired will be recommended following a description of the two main types of aphasia.

1. *Expressive Aphasia*

Expressive aphasia is characterized by an inability to express oneself due to brain damage. This may occur as the result of a stroke or a progressive dementia. Associated features of an expressive aphasia include restricted output of language and dysarthria, that is, difficulty in speech production due to unco-ordinated muscles of the speech apparatus. While the individual comprehends written and verbal instructions, retains a vocabulary, and knows the names of objects, frequently there is significant difficulty in self-expression. The effort required by the aphasic individual to communicate with others may result in intense frustration and anger.

2. *Receptive Aphasia*

This form of aphasia is characterized by a loss of comprehension. The individual can hear, but the information is improperly processed. The individual's speech may sound normal, is produced with little effort, and the grammar is usually intact; however, the content produced is frequently meaningless. Reading and writing skills may also be impaired. The individual is often unaware of the impairment and therefore is usually less frustrated than the expressive aphasic. The use of pictures, photographs, and gestures may be of help in communicating with the receptive aphasic.

Guidelines for Communicating with the Mentally Impaired Elderly

1. Approach the individual in a calm friendly manner. Always identify yourself, and stand in front of the individual in order to obtain eye contact. Take the individual's hand, and address by name.
2. Pace the conversation, as the individual has a short attention span and fatigues easily.
3. Allow increased time for the individual to respond. Encourage and support all attempts at speaking. Avoid correcting mistakes by restating what you thought the message was.
4. Reduce or eliminate competing background noises.
5. Keep the message simple, and speak slowly but naturally. Accompany verbal communication with appropriate non-verbal cues or signals. Use pictures or gestures to get the message across.
6. Ask only one question at a time. Wait for a response before asking another. If the individual does not respond, ask the question in exactly the same way.
7. It is most important to recognize the individual's emotional/mental state, for example, frustration, depression, or hostility.
8. Aim to reduce anxiety by reassuring the individual. Professionals should have a mental readiness to listen.
9. Seek clarification from the individual to be sure the message has been understood correctly.
10. Always assess for other sensory losses, such as hearing and vision.

The essential components of effective communication involve active listening, respect, and genuine interest. The professional helper must modify the approach according to the elder person's specific capabilities.

CONCLUSION

Throughout this chapter, behavioral management strategies for the mentally impaired elderly have been presented. The approaches recommended will enhance the quality of life for both the elderly relative and caregiver. Many of the strategies suggested are applicable to professional and family caregivers committed to the challenge of community-based care.

REFERENCES AND SUGGESTED READINGS

Barrol M. A. 1980. "Psychosocial Aspects of Incontinence in the Aged Person." *Psychosocial Nursing: Care of the Aged.* Ed. I. M. Burnside. New York: McGraw-Hill.

Eisdorfer C. 1980. "Paranoia and Schizophrenia—Disorders in Later Life." *Handbook of Geriatric Psychiatry.* Ed. Busse and Blazer. New York: Van Nostrand Reinhold.

Highway Traffic Act. 1980. Chapter 198. Section 177. Revised Statutes of Ontario.

Hussain R. A. and R. Davis. 1985. *Responsive Care: Behavioral Interventions with Elderly Persons.* Illinois: Research Press.

Le Riche H. W. 1980. "Some Simple Facts About Urinary Incontinence in the Elderly." *Canadian Family Physician.* 26: 99.

Mace N. and P. V. Rabins. 1981. *The Thirty-Six Hour Day.* Baltimore: The Johns Hopkins University Press.

Ouslander J. G., R. L. Kane and I.B. Abrass. September 10/1982. "Urinary Incontinence in Elderly Nursing Home Patients." *Journal of the American Medical Association.* No. 10. 248: 1194.

Rabins P.V., N. Mace and M. J. Lucas. July 1982. "The Impact of Dementia on the Family." *Journal of the American Medical Association.* 248: 333.

Rader J. and J. Doan. July 1985. "How to Decrease Wandering, A Form of Agenda Behaviour." *Geriatric Nursing.* 6: 198.

Raskind M. and M. Storrie. 1980. "Organic Mental Disorders." *Handbook of Geriatric Psychiatry.* Ed. Busse and Blazer. New York: Van Nostrand Reinhold.

Verwoerdt A. 1981. *Clinical Geropsychiatry.* 2nd ed. Baltimore: Williams and Wilkins.

Williams M. E. and F. C. Pannill. January 1980. "Urinary Incontinence in the Elderly." *Canadian Family Physician.* 26: 895.

11

Medication

Barry A. Martin, M.D., F.R.C.P.(C)

Medication is required for the effective treatment of specific symptoms and behavior which present during the course of some mental disorders in the geriatric population. The various symptoms of depression are those most commonly in need of drug treatment because of their severity, duration, and frequency in the population. Also very common are symptoms of anxiety and insomnia which may occur alone or as part of a syndrome such as depression or dementia. Much less commonly encountered are the persecutory ideas and delusions, agitation and aggression of the paranoid disorders and dementia.

The prescription of medication to geriatric patients is complicated by the physiological changes which occur with advancing age and the frequent presence of concurrent physical illnesses. The prescription of psychopharmaceuticals may be further complicated by those symptoms of mental disorder which impair cognitive functioning and, thus, compromise the appropriate use of medication.

This chapter addresses the common problems encountered and the general principles to be followed in prescribing medication for the elderly. Clinical protocols for the use of the major groups of psychopharmaceutical agents are presented. In addition, the biochemistry and mechanism of action of the antidepressants and major tranquillizers are summarized to facilitate understanding of their side effects and the rationale for their use.

COMMON PROBLEMS AND GENERAL PRINCIPLES OF GERIATRIC PHARMACOLOGY

Physiological Changes of Ageing

Advancing age is associated with a number of physiological changes which directly affect the response to drugs. The net effect of these changes is a higher plasma concentration and increased responsiveness to drugs for any given dosage compared to younger adults.

Diminished lean body mass, total body water, and plasma volume produce increased serum drug concentrations. Diminished plasma protein binding further increases the concentration of free or active drug in the serum. An increase in body fat may also lead to an accumulation of fat-soluble drugs. These factors are particularly relevant to most psychotropic drugs which are both fat-soluble and highly bound to plasma proteins. In general, the sensitivity of drug receptors in various target organs is increased leading to a greater responsiveness to drugs.

The greatest single factor contributing to the increased serum concentration of drugs is the dramatic decline in renal function with age. Creatinine clearance may be reduced by one-third because of decreased glomerular filtration and tubular excretion. At the same time, serum creatinine may be normal because the decreased lean body mass produces less creatinine.

Changes in gastrointestinal physiology and liver function may decrease the absorption or increase the plasma half-life of drugs. However, these are not as directly age related as the previously noted changes.

It must be noted that these physiological changes may increase not only the therapeutic or target effects of drugs but also their side effects. Homeostasis (physiological stability) is impaired in the elderly such that they are more vulnerable to drug-induced postural hypotension. The presence of degenerative diseases of the brain may also increase the vulnerability of the central nervous system to the side effects of the psychotropic drugs. In general terms, the elderly are most vulnerable to the following common side effects of the psychotropic drugs: sedation and related effects, extrapyramidal motor symptoms, hypotension, cardiac conduction defects, and anticholinergic effects. (These are described later in this chapter.)

This altered physiology has several important implications in prescribing for the elderly. The first principle is that geriatric patients are not old adults just as pediatric patients are not small adults. Their unique physiology demands more careful attention to drug dosages and serum concentrations. As a general rule, initial drug dosages should be low and titrated upwards to therapeutic levels. When available, serum drug concentrations should be monitored. It must be remembered that patients who have been maintained on medication to treat a chronic illness may require progressively lower dosages to maintain the same serum level as they age.

The function of relevant metabolic and excretory pathways should be screened prior to prescribing a drug. It is particularly important to adjust the dosage of renally excreted drugs according to the creatinine clearance rather than serum creatinine. [Creatinine clearance $= (140–age) \times$ weight (kg)/72 $\times$ serum creatinine]

Concurrent Diseases, Polypharmacy, and Adverse Drug Reactions

The ageing process almost invariably includes the acquisition of one or more chronic diseases and an increased susceptiblity to acute illnesses. Thus, geriatric patients with mental disorders very often have concurrent diseases for which drugs may have been prescribed. (While those over 65 years of age constitute only 10 percent of the total population, they receive over 25 percent of all prescription drugs, averaging three or four per person.) In addition, over-the-counter and home remedies for ubiquitous aches and pains, constipation, and insomnia are used much more frequently by the elderly than by younger adults.

"Polypharmacy" is the generic term for the many patterns of multiple drug use. It often has a pejorative connotation, implying that the drug taking and prescribing are both unnecessary and inappropriate medical practice. While that may be true in many cases, the elderly as a group do have a legitimate need for more medical treatment, including drugs, than other segments of the population. The more usual pathway to polypharmacy is through well-intentioned attempts to find a pharmacological remedy for all the physical problems of ageing. As the elderly accumulate symptoms, they may also accumulate drugs.

It is useful to conceptualize the many physical, psychological, and social variables that influence the extent to which people seek medical care. These variables in turn influence physicians' responses, including the prescription of drugs.

The number and persistence of symptoms, their perceived seriousness, and the resultant social and physical disability are the initial determinants of a decision to seek medical care. The ability and inclination to recognize and respond to symptoms are influenced by past experience with illness, available information and medical knowledge, by the cultural/familial emphasis on tolerance or stoicism, and other personality traits. The extent to which medical care is actually sought out is greatly influenced by its availability and accessibility.

In this broad context, a number of factors may contribute to multiple drug use. In general, the elderly have, or are at risk of, more diseases than younger adults. As a result, they may be more preoccupied with their health; more symptoms may be taken seriously and presenting complaints to physicians may be more persistent. Underlying mental disorders may be translated into physical symptoms. A drug may be correctly prescribed but continued unnecessarily after the presenting problem has resolved because the elderly patient and/or the physician assume the condition to be chronic and in need of sustained drug management. With unlimited availability of physicians, patients may receive medication unknown to others who are also prescribing for them. Alternatively, drug treatment for a specific problem may be initiated by a specialist with follow-up by a general practitioner who may be reluctant to discontinue the drug if uncertain of the original indications. (It should also be noted that many elderly patients under report symptoms as a result of, for example, an increased pain threshold or denial of illness. This may lead to under-utilization of medical services, including drugs.)

The combination of polypharmacy and altered physiology renders the elderly more vulnerable to adverse drug reactions. Such reactions may be the result of the therapeutic effect, side effects or toxicity of a drug, or untoward interactions between drugs. Among the drugs most commonly prescribed for the elderly are digoxin, thiazide diuretics, oral hypoglycemics, anti-hypertensives, antibiotics, antidepressants, and minor tranquillizers. Most of the common adverse drug reactions in the elderly involve these medications alone or in combination with other drugs as summarized in Table 11.1.

TABLE 11.1

Common Adverse Drug Reactions in the Elderly

Drug	Adverse Reaction
1. Digoxin	Increased toxicity. Potentiated by hypokalemia induced by potassium—depleting diuretics (i.e. hydrochlorothiazide, furosemide).
2. Antihypertensives	Hypotension and postural hypotension. Potentiated by tricyclic antidepressants (i.e. amitriptyline), neuroleptics (i.e. chlorpromazine), diuretics, levodopa, anticholinergics (i.e. benztropine mesylate, procyclidine HCl).
3. Anticholinergics (Antiparkinsonian)	Increased peripheral and central anticholinergic effects (dry mouth, decreased visual accommodation, tachycardia, urinary retention, constipation; drowsiness, confusion, agitation, delirium, visual hallucinations). Potentiated by tricyclic antidepressants, neuroleptics.
4. Lithium	Increased toxicity. Potentiated by diuretics which increase lithium reabsorption.
5. Major Tranquillizers (Neuroleptics)	Increased sensitivity to sedating, extrapyramidal, and anticholinergic side effects. Potentiated by tricyclic antidepressants and anticholinergics.
6. Tricyclic Antidepressants	Increased sensitivity to sedating, anticholinergic, and cardiovascular (varying degrees of heart block) side effects. Potentiated by neuroleptics and anticholinergics.
7. Benzodiazepines	Increased sedation due to tissue accumulation of long-acting agents (i.e. diazepam, flurazepam). Potentiated by alcohol and neuroleptics.

A number of general principles for prescribing medication for the elderly have been derived from the aforementioned patient, physician, and drug interactions. These principles may be summarized as follows:

1. A very detailed medication history should be obtained from the patient and/or informant. All prescription and non-prescription drugs, alcohol, tobacco, and caffeine should be included. All medication should be made available for inspection to determine the dates and quantities of the prescriptions and the names of all prescribing physicians. Enquiry should be made of the dosage, schedule of administration, regularity of use, and the reason for using each drug. In so doing, an attempt should be made to determine whether or not a drug is used to treat the symptoms for which it was originally prescribed. Alternatively, the use of the drug may have become habitual or a remedy for entirely different symptoms. Patients should be asked if they share medications that have been prescribed for another person. It should be determined whether or not the patient can read and understand the relevant instructions on medication containers. (While taking such a history, the competence of the patient to self-administer medication can be assessed.)

2. On the basis of the complete history, physical and mental status examinations, and relevant ancillary tests, all unnecessary medication should be discontinued. The patient should be encouraged to discard the unnecessary drugs in the presence of a physician.
3. Regimens for necessary drugs should be simplified and the need for each drug should be reviewed periodically.
4. The duration of treatment should be specified.
5. Treatment priorities should be established to avoid the prescription of drugs for all presenting problems.
6. When choices are available, psychopharmaceuticals with the least sedative, anticholinergic and hypotensive side effects should be used.

Further prescribing guidelines are presented in the sections on non-compliance and specific drug groups.

Non-Compliance

When patients have been prescribed appropriate drugs in correct dosages, non-compliance may lead to ineffective treatment outcomes and/or adverse drug reactions. Non-compliance refers to the failure to take medications according to instructions and includes never having the prescription filled, premature discontinuation, using an incorrect dosage (too high or low) or dosage schedule, and taking the drug for the wrong indication.

The rates of non-compliance by the elderly usually range in the order of 25 to 60 percent of patients. While the definition and measurement of non-compliance varies, the consistently high reported rates lead to the conclusion that it cannot be assumed that patients follow medication instructions. Non-compliance rates for psychotropic drugs are not always higher than those for other drug groups. Rates for the elderly are not always higher than those for younger adults although the elderly more often present with some of the specific problems leading to non-compliance.

There are many reasons for non-compliance by elderly patients including specific physical and cognitive impairments and polypharmacy. Others are related to the variables that affect patients' decisions to seek medical care as described previously. Non-compliant patients may perceive themselves less threatened by illness and may have less concern with their health. In the face of severe symptoms, frank denial of illness may lead to non-compliance. Related to this are patients' general attitudes and beliefs about disease and the relative benefit of drugs versus tincture of time. Scepticism about the value of medication may prevail even in the presence of severe illness.

Anything that interferes with understanding the illness and the reasons for using medication may decrease compliance. This is particularly relevant for elderly patients with mental disorders; an impaired mental status may preclude adequate understanding of medication instructions.

The extent to which the side effects of medication and dosage schedules disrupt daily living are important determinants of compliance. The severe side effects of some psychotropic drugs may be more troublesome to the patient than the symptoms for which the drugs have been prescribed. This is particularly true for asymptomatic patients who have been prescribed maintenance/pro-phylactic drugs.

Compliance decreases as the number of medications increases because it is more difficult to comprehend and organize the daily dosages and schedules. This is particularly true for newly prescribed medication when dosages must be changed frequently to reach therapeutic levels.

Compliance may be decreased by any difficulty encountered in obtaining the medication, opening the container, swallowing the drug, or identifying the drug among others that have been prescribed. (A number of elderly patients dump all their medication into one container.)

A number of general principles should be followed to improve compliance by elderly patients. This should be regarded as a very high priority in overall patient management with the devotion of sufficient time. Again, it may not be assumed that patients will comply in faith with their physicians' instructions. These principles may be summarized as follows:

1. Patients do not require a complete understanding of the pathophysiology and pharmacology of his/her illness. However, sufficient information should be provided to ensure that the patient has a rationale for taking medication as instructed. Information about side effects must be presented to avoid undue alarm and non-compliance when they occur.

2. The patient's responsibility for compliance should be addressed directly. It should be noted that failure to comply precludes an accurate assessment of the effectiveness or failure of treatment which in turn may interfere with the choice of alternative management plans.

3. The potential benefits and limitations of the drug should be explained so that the patient has appropriate expectations. Parenthetically, these instructions are in keeping with present standards of disclosure for obtaining informed consent to treatment. Supplementary written information may be useful.

4. Insofar as possible, medication regimens should be simplified. Once a day dosages should be used when appropriate for any given drug and more than three times a day schedules should be avoided. (Almost all psycho-pharmaceuticals are effective when administered once a day.) Specific times of administration should be established to minimize disruption of the patient's usual daily activities. Clear verbal and written instructions should be provided regarding the dosages and duration of treatment. Therefore, prescription medication should not be labelled "as directed".

5. Accessibility to the medication must be ensured. Patients should be assessed to determine whether or not decreased strength, arthritic pain, impaired co-ordination, or mental confusion interfere with opening childproof containers. Capsules or liquid medication should be prescribed if dysphagia occurs with tablets. If visual acuity is impaired, medications of similar size, shape and color should be avoided and generic equivalents dispensed. (For example, some digoxin tablets are almost identical to some anticho-linergic tablets used to manage the extrapyramidal side effects of major tranquillizers.) Daily dosage dispensing trays should be used when indicated. Patients may form an association between the color or shape of a pill and

its indication. This may be disrupted when generic equivalents are substituted. Therefore, the drug preparation should not be altered during the course of treatment.

6. Compliance should be assessed routinely and adequate follow-up appointments provided. As previously noted, patients should be asked to describe when and how they are taking their medication. Pills should be counted and blood levels should be obtained periodically. Patterns of "lost" prescriptions or premature renewals should be investigated.

7. Whenever possible, the medication history should be confirmed by an informant. For many elderly patients, compliance can be ensured only through adequate supervision.

Physician non-compliance must also be considered, particularly in the treatment of mental disorders. General practitioners and non-psychiatric specialists are often reluctant to prescribe psychotropic drugs in adequate therapeutic dosages. This issue is addressed further in the following section.

Inadequate Therapeutic Trials of Medication

While the tolerance for usual adult dosages of drugs is decreased in the elderly, dosages must be sufficient to obtain therapeutic blood levels. When drug treatment is indicated, the prescription of subtherapeutic or homeopathic dosages is unacceptable. For example, it is not uncommon for elderly depressed patients to be treated with dosages of tricyclic antidepressants in the order of 10 to 30 mg per day. These dosages are harmful because they are almost always ineffective. Having prescribed antidepressants, the patient is offered some hope for recovery. Antidepressant drugs in therapeutic dosages often do not take effect for three or four weeks. Prolonging this interval without improvement by using subtherapeutic dosages may accentuate the depressive symptom of hopelessness. Further, it may discredit psychiatric intervention so that the patient does not seek more appropriate treatment.

The general principle to be followed is that drugs are to be prescribed cautiously to the elderly but the treatment should be vigorous with adequate dosages. Similarly, therapeutic dosages must be administered over a sufficiently long interval to ensure that an adequate trial has been given. Otherwise, the incorrect conclusion may be drawn that the drug is ineffective resulting in its premature discontinuation. This error may be compounded when less effective alternatives are prescribed.

MECHANISM OF ACTION OF PSYCHOTROPIC DRUGS

In general, the drugs used to treat mental disorders in the elderly exert both their therapeutic effects and common side effects by influencing the function of neurotransmitters in the brain and in the autonomic nervous system. [Neurotransmitters are a number of chemicals which are synthesized and stored in neurons (nerve cells); each neuron produces one neurotransmitter. When a neuron discharges electrically, a small amount of its transmitter is released into the narrow spaces (synapses) between adjacent neurons. The neurotransmitter crosses the synapses to stimulate chemical receptors on adjacent neurons leading to their discharge. In this way, "messages" are transmitted from cell to cell in the nervous system. The concentration of the neurotransmitters varies within the nervous system. Therefore, a drug predominantly affecting one neurotransmitter will have its principal effect on the areas of highest concentration of that transmitter. The neurotransmitters in the brain that are implicated in most current theories about the chemical causes of mental disorders are the catecholamines (dopamine and norepinephrine), serotonin, and acetylcholine. The neurotransmitters in the autonomic nervous system are epinephrine and acetylcholine.]

In brief, the psychotropic drugs used to treat the elderly act in a number of ways to increase or decrease the amounts of certain neurotransmitters that are functionally available to receptors. Some of the drugs occupy receptors to block the access of transmitters and, hence, to prevent nerve cells from discharging. Others mimic neurotransmitters to stimulate receptors and others increase the concentration of transmitters by preventing their inactivation. Much of the effect of drugs is due to their structural similarity to various neuro-transmitters, illustrated in Figure 11.1. (The groups of drugs illustrated are discussed in ensuing sections.) That similarity to the naturally occurring chemicals permits drugs to interact with receptors in a manner analogous to the fit between a lock and key. What appear to be minor structural differences between drugs may result in very substantial differences in their therapeutic and side effects. On the other hand, similarity of the chemical ring and side-chain structure among different groups of drugs may lead to very similar side effects. The therapeutic mechanisms of action and side effects of specific groups of drugs are presented in the ensuing sections.

TRICYCLIC ANTIDEPRESSANTS AND MONOAMINE OXIDASE INHIBITORS

Clinical Indications

The majority of elderly patients who present with symptoms of depression have relatively mild disorders which do not require treatment with antidepressant drugs. Patients with a lifelong history of labile moodiness, pessimism, hypo-chondriasis or other personality traits similar to depressive symptoms are unlikely to respond to antidepressants. Patients experiencing acute bereavement or other life crises may present with more severe symptoms of depression but which are usually self-limiting over a few weeks or months. These conditions are most effectively managed with psychotherapy, social support, and/or environmental changes to resolve the identified problems.

Antidepressants should be reserved for cases of moderate and severe depression. Determination of the severity of depression requires a clinical judgment based upon the constellation of presenting symptoms, their intensity, and the duration of the illness. The symptoms of severe depression may be summarized as follows: depressed mood and anhedonia; feelings of self-worthlessness and guilt; hopelessness for the future; mood-congruent delusions;

FIGURE 11.1
The Chemical Structure of Neurotransmitters and Psychotropic Drugs

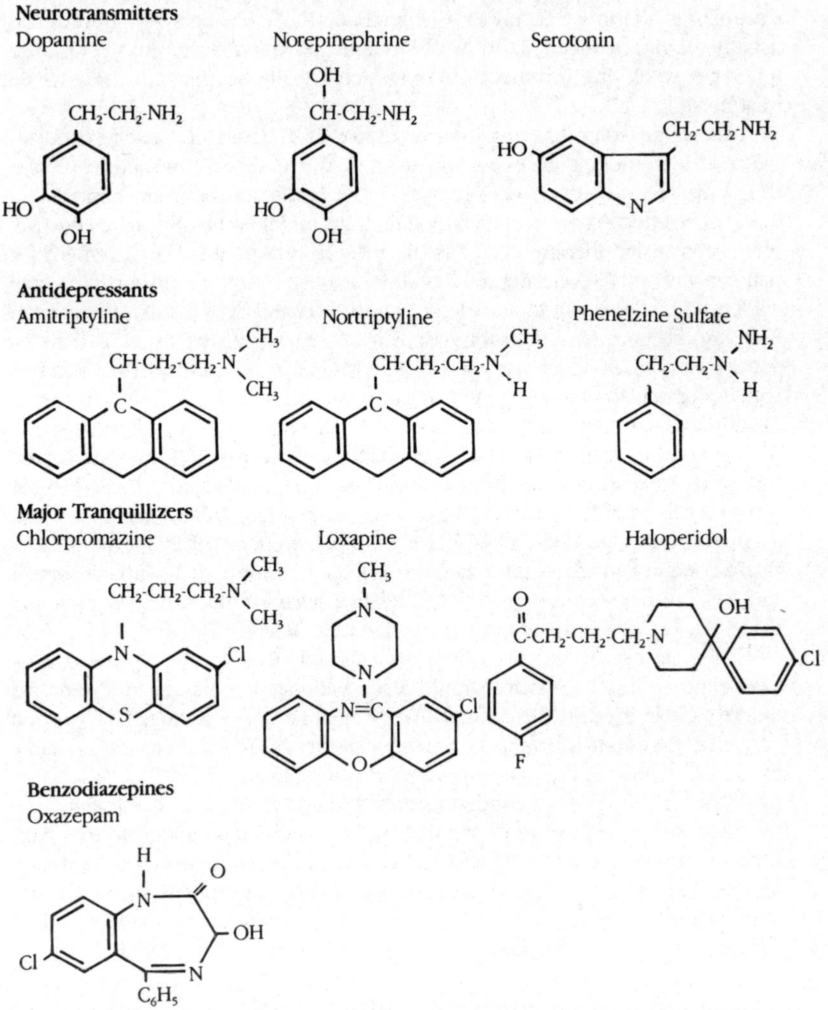

Neurotransmitters
Dopamine   Norepinephrine   Serotonin

Antidepressants
Amitriptyline   Nortriptyline   Phenelzine Sulfate

Major Tranquillizers
Chlorpromazine   Loxapine   Haloperidol

Benzodiazepines
Oxazepam

"endogenous" symptoms of psychomotor retardation or agitation and loss of sleep, appetite, weight, and libido; and active suicidal ideation with a planned and available means or attempted suicide with lethal intent. Some elderly patients with quite severe depression may also present with somatic complaints which dominate the clinical picture. Patients with depression secondary to severe illness (i.e. stroke or dementia) may also require treatment with antidepressants.

[Electroconvulsive therapy (ECT) is a commonly used form of treatment for patients with moderate to severe depression. Despite many concerns about its side effects, the treatment as presently administered does not cause permanent memory loss for new information (anterograde amnesia) and does not cause structural brain damage (loss of neurons). Almost all patients who receive the treatment experience a patchy loss of memory for some events immediately preceding and during the course of treatment (retrograde amnesia). Each treatment is administered under a general anesthetic. Patients with depression usually require between six to twelve treatments which are given two or three times per week. Improvement of depression usually begins after three to six treatments.

There are some specific indications for ECT based on its effectiveness, the onset of its therapeutic effect, and its safety. Currently available antidepressant drugs may require three or four weeks before the onset of an appreciable therapeutic effect. Therefore, even though drugs might eventually prove effective, electroconvulsive therapy (ECT) is the most appropriate initial treatment for patients with very severe depression and for those running a malignant course evidenced by the intent to suicide or by inanition and dehydration. Depression with mood-congruent delusions is also more responsive to ECT than to antidepressants alone or in combination with major tranquillizers. For patients with recurrent severe depression, previously unresponsive to adequate trials of antidepressants, ECT is the treatment of choice rather than to prolong suffering during a further drug trial with a low probability of success. ECT is also indicated for severe depression when antidepressants are contraindicated, when adequate serum levels cannot be achieved because of intolerable side effects, or when their risks outweigh those of ECT. For example, a course of ECT may be safer than a course of antidepressant medication for a geriatric patient with concurrent cardiovascular disease because of the relative safety of modern anesthesia and electrocardiographic monitoring during the treatment.]

The majority of patients who are moderately to severely depressed and/ or previously drug responsive should receive adequate trials of antidepressants before ECT is used as the second line of treatment. A substantial proportion of such patients may prove to be unresponsive to drugs but there is no reliable means of identifying the non-responders in advance.

One of the tricyclic antidepressants should be used as the initial drug treatment for most cases of depression in the elderly. If an adequate trial fails, another tricyclic should be tried. A monamine oxidase inhibitor (MAOI) should be considered only when depression has been refractory to tricyclic anti-depressants or when an atypical clinical picture is dominated by anxiety, social phobia, and somatic complaints.

Therapeutic Mechanism of Action

The therapeutic mechanisms of action of the antidepressants are related to contemporary theories about the biological etiology of depression. In general terms, these theories postulate that depression is caused by or associated with a decrease in neurotransmitters that are functionally active in synapses in the brain. Current theories suggest that the neurotransmitters which are deficient in depression are serotonin and/or norepinephrine.

FIGURE 11.2

Therapeutic Mechanism of Action of the Tricyclic Antidepressants and Monoamine Oxidase Inhibitors

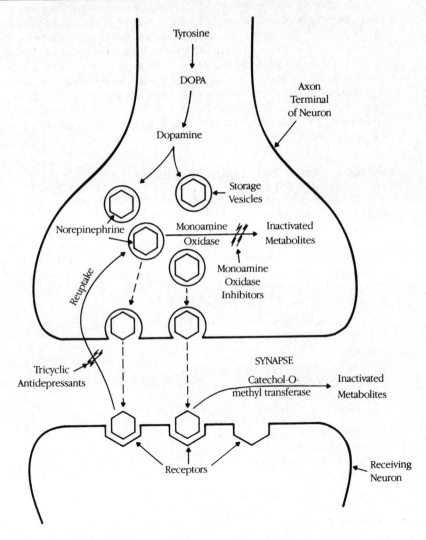

The therapeutic mechanisms of action of the tricyclic antidepressants and the MAOI's are presented in Figure 11.2. The metabolism of norepinephrine is illustrated and the drugs have a similar effect on serotonin. Norepinephrine is synthesized from the amino acid tyrosine through a series of chemical reactions inside nerve cells. The norepinephrine is stored in vesicles which form a circulating pool of transmitter in the neuron. When the neuron discharges, some norepinephrine is released into the synapses where it reacts with receptors to stimulate adjacent neurons. The transmitter is then released from the receptor sites and inactivated in a number of ways. A small amount is metabolized in the synapse by the enzyme catechol-O-methyltransferase. Most of the transmitter is re-absorbed by the neuron in which it was synthesized. It then reenters the transmitter pool in the neuron where it may be reused or metabolized by the enzyme monoamine oxidase. The tricyclic antidepressants block the re-absorption or reuptake of norepinephrine and serotonin and, thus, increase their concentration at receptor sites. As their name suggests, the MAOI's decrease the inactivation of norepinephrine and serotonin by inhibiting the enzyme monoamine oxidase. Thus, the anti-depressants increase the amount of neuro-transmitters by decreasing their inactivation. It should also be noted that the central anticholinergic effects of the antidepressants may contribute to their therapeutic action.

Adverse Effects and Contraindications

The most common and potential adverse effects of the tricyclic antide-pressants are summarized in Table 11.2. The potential adverse effects of MAOI's are similar. The potential benefit of prescribing a drug must be considered in relation to the risk of these adverse effects and their potential to exacerbate concurrent diseases. Fortunately, the severe and/or dangerous adverse reactions are very rare.

TABLE 11.2

Potential Adverse Effects of Tricyclic Antidepressants

Anticholinergic Effects

1. Brain: mild confusion to delirium
2. Eyes: impaired accommodation with blurred vision; increased intra-ocular pressure (exacerbation of open and narrow angle glaucoma)
3. Cardiovascular system: tachycardia; postural hypotension
4. Gastrointestinal tract: dry mouth; nausea; dyspepsia; impaired motility (constipation to paralytic ileus); cholestatic jaundice
5. Genitourinary tract: urinary retention; impotence
6. Skin: increased perspiration

Other Effects on the Brain

1. Sedation or stimulation (increased or decreased sleep)
2. Extrapyramidal symptoms: tremor; rigidity; akathisia
3. Decreased seizure threshold
4. Incoordination; ataxia

Other Effects

1. Cardiovascular system: cardiac conduction defects with varying degrees of heart block and increased vulnerability to ectopic beats; T-wave flattening and inversion
2. Hemopoietic: bone marrow suppression
3. Skin: allergic rashes; pruritis; photosensitivity
4. Endocrine: decreased blood sugar with increased appetite and weight gain

Tricyclic antidepressants should not be used by patients recovering from a myocardial infarct or by those with acute congestive heart failure. They should be used with caution in patients with cardiac arrhythmias and conduction defects. Because of their anticholinergic side effects, they are contraindicated in the presence of untreated/undiagnosed glaucoma, paralytic ileus, and severe urinary retention. They are contraindicated in patients with a known hypersensitivity or allergy to them. Severely suicidal patients should not be given access to more than a one week supply of a tricyclic antidepressant.

The MAOI's must be used cautiously in patients with concurrent cardio-vascular disease because they commonly produce hypotension or hypertension. They are absolutely contraindicated in combination with certain foods, beverages, and drugs which may precipitate a hypertensive crisis. When prescribed, patients must be given a list and instructed to avoid those substances which include the following: other antidepressants, over-the-counter cold, hay fever and weight reduction medication; coffee, tea and cola drinks in excess; alcohol; cheese, sour cream, chicken and beef liver, chocolate, yeast extract, broad beans, pickled herring, oxo, bovril, marmite, raisins, and soy sauce.

Treatment Protocol

To date, the claims of a more rapid onset of therapeutic effect and fewer significant side effects for new antidepressant drugs has not been established for geriatric patients. (Such claims must be interpreted cautiously because clinical trials preceding the marketing of new drugs often do not include a sufficient number of elderly patients.) In addition, no one tricyclic antidepressant has been found to be more effective than all others. Therefore, the choice of drugs for geriatric patients is largely dependent upon their side effects.

Nortriptyline is recommended as the antidepressant of first choice in the geriatric population for a number of reasons. At therapeutic dosages, it has been found to have relatively few clinically significant effects on the heart and blood pressure. It is not as sedating or stimulating as several other antidepressants. Further, the range of therapeutic blood levels has been established such that the dosage can be monitored.

Although doxepin hydrochloride is often recommended for this age group, claims for fewer cardiovascular side effects have not been substantiated at equivalent therapeutic dosages. At present, it is recommended as a second choice. Amitriptyline should not be used because of its higher frequency of cardiovascular and sedating side effects when prescribed in therapeutic dosages. (Amitriptyline is metabolized to nortriptyline in the body. Despite their structural similarity, there is considerable difference in their side effects. See Figure 11.1).

A suggested routine protocol for prescribing nortriptyline to geriatric patients is presented in Table 11.3. This should be modified as clinically indicated (i.e. slower and smaller dosage increases in the presence of troublesome side effects)

Anticholinergic and sedating side effects are prominent from the onset of treatment and may gradually decrease. The therapeutic effect usually begins after one to three weeks of a therapeutic dose. Initial signs of response may

TABLE 11.3

Clinical Protocol for Prescribing Nortriptyline to Geriatric Patients

1. Pre-treatment EKG. (Serial EKG's at successive dosage increases as clinically indicated.) Pre-treatment screening of renal, hepatic, and hemopoietic function.

2. Initial dose: 25 mg per day for 3 days.

3. Increase dose by 25 mg per day every 2 to 4 days up to 100 mg per day.

4. Dosage schedule: b.i.d. or h.s. depending upon side effects.

5. Blood level: maintain on 100 mg per day for 5 days (75 mg if side effects are severe) and obtain blood level. Therpeutic levels are between 50 and 150 ng/mL.

6. Adjust dose to maintain blood levels in the upper part of the therapeutic range. The usual therapeutic dose range is 75 to 150 mg per day.

7. Continue therapeutic dose for **at least 4 to 6 weeks** even if there is no apparent response.

---

be improved sleep, and increased energy and activity (or decreased agitation). *Subjective improvement in mood may not occur for several more weeks. Cognitive symptoms of impaired self-esteem and future orientation may be the last to recover.* (The therapeutic response to a MAOI is similar.)

The full therapeutic dose should be continued four to eight weeks after recovery. It should then be reduced to a maintenance level (50 to 75 mg per day) for three to six months to prevent relapse. The dosages and duration vary depending upon the severity of illness, the time required for a therapeutic response, and the past history of relapse.

It should be noted that the placebo effect and concurrent psychotherapy/ social support may contribute substantially to the therapeutic effects of the antidepressants in a large proportion of patients.

If there is no clinical response after an adequate therapeutic trial of at least four to six weeks, a second tricyclic antidepressant should be tried with a protocol similar to that previously described. A tricyclic from a different chemical group may be considered (i.e. clomipramine hydrochloride). Patients who remain refractory should be referred for psychiatric consultation. At that time, MAOI's (i.e. phenelzine sulfate) or various drug combinations may be considered.

LITHIUM CARBONATE

Clinical Indications

Lithium carbonate is most commonly prescribed to geriatric patients who have a long history of bipolar affective disorder. (This is also called manic-depressive disorder. Patients who are treated with lithium usually have a history of episodes of both depression and mania or hypomania. The latter are characterized by an irritable or euphoric mood, increased motor activity, increased rate of thinking and speech, and impaired social judgment.) While lithium may be used to treat acute episodes of mania or hypomania, these are relatively uncommon in the geriatric population. Lithium is more often used to prevent relapses of mania and depression. As such, it is prescribed continuously over long periods of time.

Lithium may also be prescribed as an adjunct to tricyclic antidepressants in the management of refractory depression.

Adverse Effects and Contraindications

Lithium carbonate is a salt which is excreted by the kidneys in a manner similar to that for sodium. Approximately 80 percent is re-absorbed in the proximal tubules such that only 20 percent is excreted with each passage through the kidneys. As the sodium concentration in the blood decreases, more lithium is re-absorbed in the kidneys. In addition, the lithium concentration at any given dosage increases as the creatinine clearance decreases. Therefore, the elderly are particularly vulnerable to the accumulation of excessive serum concentrations. The range of serum levels within which lithium can be administered safely is quite narrow such that careful management is required to prevent toxicity.

The adverse effects of lithium are presented in Table 11.4. The contraindications are relative to the risks of those adverse effects and the exacerbation of concurrent diseases. Lithium must be used cautiously when there is a risk of sodium depletion (i.e. diuretics, excessive sweating, dietary restriction).

TABLE 11.4
Potential Adverse Effects of Lithium Carbonate

Common Side Effects
1. Central nervous system: fine tremor of the hands; fatigue
2. Cardiovascular system: T-wave flattening and inversion
3. Gastrointestinal tract: dry mouth; nausea; loose stools; abdominal pain
4. Genitourinary tract: polyuria; thirst
5. Hemopoietic: leukocytosis
6. Endocrine: impaired release of thyroid hormone with goitre; edema; weight gain

Signs of Toxicity
1. Central nervous system: coarse tremor, muscle twitching and hyperreflexia, episodic rigidity; over-sedation, confusion, restlessness, stupor, coma; seizures; blurred vision; nystagmus; slurred speech; ataxia; incontinence
2. Cardiovascular system: arrhythmias; hypotension; hypertension
3. Gastrointestinal tract: increased nausea; vomiting; diarrhea

Treatment Protocol

The physiological changes of ageing, the presence of concurrent diseases, polypharmacy and non-compliance make the elderly very vulnerable to the development of lithium intoxication. Thus, very careful management is required. A suggested protocol for prescribing lithium carbonate to the elderly is presented in Table 11.5.

TABLE 11.5

Clinical Protocol for Prescribing Lithium Carbonate to Geriatric Patients

1. Pre-treatment EKG, electrolytes and screening of renal, thyroid and hemopoietic functions.

2. Initial dose: 300 mg per day for 3 days.

3. Increase dose to 600 mg per day.

4. Dosage schedule: b.i.d. or h.s. depending upon side effects.

5. Blood level: maintain on 600 mg per day for 7 days and obtain blood level. Draw blood approximately 12 hours following last lithium dose. Therapeutic levels range approximately between 0.5 and 0.8 mmol/L.

6. Adjust dose in 150 to 300 mg per day increments to obtain therapeutic levels. Maintain each dose for 7 days and obtain blood level before dose change. The usual therapeutic dose range is 600 to 900 mg per day.

7. Blood level: one week after each subsequent dose change; whenever sodium may be depleted (diuretics, sweating, dietary restriction, vomiting, severe diarrhea); whenever intoxication is suspected; whenever there is a recurrence of mania or depression; routinely every 6 to 12 months.

8. Electrolytes and screening of renal and thyroid function every 6 to 12 months.

It must be noted that lithium toxicity is most likely at serum levels above 2 mmol/L in young adults. In the elderly, it may occur at much lower levels. The range of 0.5 to 0.8 mmol/L is suggested as a prophylactic level and as an adjunct to tricyclic antidepressants. Higher levels may be required to treat acute manic symptoms.

Patients who have been maintained on lithium since younger adulthood will require progressively lower dosages to maintain therapeutic blood levels as they age.

MAJOR TRANQUILLIZERS (NEUROLEPTICS)

Clinical Indications

The geriatric population is well past the age of onset of most of the mental disorders for which the major tranquillizers or neuroleptics are the treatment of choice. Thus, symptoms of acute schizophrenia, schizophreniform psychoses and mania are relatively uncommon in this age group. When they do occur, major tranquillizers are indicated.

More commonly encountered are paranoid symptoms of suspiciousness and persecutory delusions with resultant irritability and/or aggressive behavior.

These symptoms may present alone as a distinct paranoid disorder or as part of the clinical picture of other mental disorders such as depression, dementia, and late onset paraphrenia. When severe, such paranoid symptoms may require treatment with major tranquillizers, often in conjunction with other forms of management for the underlying disorder.

During the course of dementia, many patients develop a very labile affect resulting in unpredictable and often unprovoked episodes of anxiety, agitation, excitement, irritability, anger, and aggressive behavior. Patients may also develop a reversal of the sleep-wakefulness cycle with agitation and restless wandering at night. A few patients have delusions and hallucinations. The neuroleptics are indicated under all of these circumstances, particularly when the behavior is dangerous to the patient or others or when it interferes substantially with other aspects of management (i.e. feeding, maintenance of hygiene).

Elderly patients with acute confusional states or delirium secondary to dementia, various physical disorders, or post-operatively may require management with neuroleptics along with more specific treatment for the underlying disorder.

Therapeutic Mechanism of Action

The principal therapeutic mechanism of action of the neuroleptics is now thought to be related to their capacity to block receptors for dopamine. Current theories suggest that some of the most florid symptoms of schizophrenia and related psychoses (i.e. delusions, hallucinations) are due to excessive amounts of dopamine in certain areas of the brain. In these areas, many of the neurons synthesize dopamine as their neurotransmitter. Both their dopamine-blocking action and their non-specific tranquillizing/sedating effect provide the rationale for using neuroleptics to treat the previously noted disorders in the elderly. (The major tranquillizers produce emotional calming, psychomotor slowing and indifference without decreasing consciousness.)

The metabolic pathways for dopamine are very similar to those illustrated for norepinephrine in Figure 11.2 earlier in this chapter. Dopamine in the storage vesicles is released into the synapses where it stimulates adjacent neurons by interacting with their receptors. The similarity of the chemical ring and side-chain structure of the neuroleptics and dopamine (illustrated in Figure 11.1 earlier in this chapter) permits the drugs to mimic dopamine and react with its receptors. In this way, the access of dopamine to the receptors is blocked such that the neurons cannot discharge. The antipsychotic potency per mg of the various neuroleptics is directly proportional to their respective dopamine-blocking capacities.

Adverse Effects and Contraindications

The potential adverse effects of the neuroleptics are summarized in Table 11.6. The most common and clinically significant side effects of these drugs are the anticholinergic and extrapyramidal.

TABLE 11.6

Potential Adverse Effects of Major Tranquillizers

Anticholinergic Effects

1. Brain: mild confusion to delirium
2. Eyes: impaired accommodation with blurred vision; increased intra-ocular pressure (exacerbation of open and narrow angle glaucoma)
3. Cardiovascular system: tachycardia; postural hypotension
4. Gastrointestinal tract: dry mouth; nausea; dyspepsia; impaired motility (constipation to paralytic ileus); cholestatic jaundice
5. Genitourinary tract: urinary retention; impotence

Other Effects on the Brain

1. Sedation and fatigue
2. Extrapyramidal syndromes
   a. Parkinsonism
   b. Akathisia
   c. Tardive dyskinesia
3. Decreased seizure threshold

Other Effects*

1. Cardiovascular system: cardiac conduction defects with varying degrees of heart block and increased vulnerability to ectopic beats; T-wave inversion
2. Hemopoietic: bone marrow suppression
3. Skin: allergic rashes; pruritus; photosensitivity
4. Endocrine: increased or decreased libido; increased appetite

---

*Extremely rare in the dosages generally prescribed to or recommended for geriatric patients

The anticholinergic effects are particularly troublesome and potentially dangerous to the elderly because of their potential to exacerbate pre-existing cardiovascular, ocular, gastrointestinal, and urinary tract disorders. In general, the severity of the anticholinergic effects of the various neuroleptics is inversely proportional to their respective dopamine-blocking capacities. That is, the neuroleptics with the least antipsychotic potency per mg have the greatest anticholinergic effects. Examples of these low potency neuroleptics are chlorpromazine, methotrimeprazine, and thioridazine.

The frequent and severe extrapyramidal effects of these drugs are due to their dopamine blockade. Dopamine is the principal neurotransmitter in the extrapyramidal motor system. [In brief, the nerve cells in this system permit the smooth initiation and even rates of contraction of skeletal muscles and their subsequent relaxation. The system operates by simultaneously relaxing and contracting opposing muscle groups. The most common disorder involving this system is Parkinson's disease. This illness develops as a result of the degeneration of nerve cells in the nigro-striatal pathway (nerve fibres passing from the substantia nigra to the putamen and caudate nucleus). The resultant dopamine deficiency leads to a tremor, muscular rigidity, and difficulty initiating voluntary movements.]

The extrapyramidal effects of the dopamine-blocking neuroleptics are very similar to the symptoms of naturally occurring Parkinson's disease. Tremor of the hands and muscular stiffness or rigidity are the most common effects. Also common is an inability to relax the muscles for prolonged periods such that patients experience a severe form of restlessness in which they report feeling compelled to keep moving. This is called akathisia.

When receptors have been blocked by neuroleptics over a prolonged period of time (usually months or years), they appear to develop an increased sensitivity to the small amounts of dopamine that pass through the blockade. This increased sensitivity (or increased number of receptors) often results in abnormal body movements called tardive dyskinesia when the neuroleptic dosage is decreased. Most commonly in the elderly, the syndrome presents as sucking and smacking movements of the lips, lateral jaw movements, puffing of the cheeks and thrusting, rolling, tremor, or fasciculations of the tongue. The syndrome may be irreversible. (A small percentage of the geriatric population has spontaneous oral movements identical to those of tardive dyskinesia.)

As might be expected, the frequency and severity of the extrapyramidal effects of the specific neuroleptics is directly proportional to their antipsychotic potency per mg and to their dopamine-blocking capacity. Examples of the high-potency neuroleptics are haloperidol, fluphenazine, trifluoperazine, and per-phenazine. In general, this group has the least anticholinergic effects.

Treatment Protocol

As a rule, the elderly are particularly sensitive to both the therapeutic and adverse effects of the neuroleptics. Therefore, for most clinical indications, the initial dosages must be very low. The choice of drug is largely determined by its principal side effects. While both anticholinergic and extrapyramidal effects are undesirable and distressing, the former may be more dangerous. Therefore, higher potency neuroleptics are generally recommended. Minimum effective dosages should be used for the shortest possible duration.

Haloperidol and loxapine are recommended for geriatric patients. Loxapine should be used when more sedation is desired. A suggested clinical protocol for their administration is presented in Table 11.7.

ANXIOLYTICS AND HYPNOTICS

Clinical Indications

Symptoms of anxiety and insomnia are extremely prevalent in the geriatric population. However, the vast majority of patients with these symptoms should not be treated with anxiolytic or hypnotic drugs. These symptoms most often occur as part of the clinical picture of other mental or physical disorders, as a result of acute or chronic social/environmental problems, or as a result of poor sleep habits and the changes in sleep physiology which occur with ageing. Under these conditions, alternative management is indicated. Unfortunately, the

TABLE 11.7

Clinical Protocol for Prescribing Haloperidol and Loxapine to Geriatric Patients

1. Initial dose:
   a. Haloperidol: 0.5 mg b.i.d.
   b. Loxapine: 5.0 mg b.i.d.
2. Increase dose every 2 to 4 days until therapeutic effect is achieved.
   a. Haloperidol: 0.5 mg per day increments
   b. Loxapine: 5.0 mg per day increments
3. Dosage schedule: b.i.d. or h.s. depending upon side effects
4. Usual therapeutic dose range
   a. Haloperidol: 1 to 5 mg per day
   b. Loxapine: 10 to 50 mg per day
5. Anticholinergic (anti-parkinsonian) drugs should be prescribed only when drug-induced extrapyramidal symptoms appear.
6. Only one neuroleptic should be prescribed at one time.

anxiolytics and hypnotics are among the drugs most over-prescribed to the elderly.

Anxiety and insomnia are often very prominent symptoms of depression. The incorrect use of anxiolytics or hypnotics may delay effective treatment with antidepressants. Similarly, anxiety/agitation and alteration of the sleep-wakefulness cycle are common features of dementia. In that syndrome, they may be more effectively managed with neuroleptics since minor tranquillizers or anxiolytics may have a disinhibiting effect on associated aggressive or impulsive behavior.

Medication should not be used as an alternative to resolving underlying social/environmental problems. In addition, medication should not necessarily be used when the source of the patient's distress is acute and self-limiting. Supportive and/or directive psychotherapy may be the most effective management.

Complaints of insomnia should be assessed carefully. Normal sleep is characterized by phasic neuromuscular activity occurring in approximately 90 min cycles. Sleep stages one, two, three and four are followed by the rapid eye movement (REM) sleep stage in which dreaming occurs. Stages one to four are characterized by progressively increasing synchronization of the electroencephalogram with increasing depth of sleep. The normal changes in physiology with advancing age include a progressive decline in REM sleep. (Infants have 50 percent REM sleep, young adults 25 percent, and the elderly 15 percent and decreasing with age.) Stages three and four (deep sleep) comprise about 20 percent of total sleep time in young adults but the elderly have virtually no stage four sleep. In addition, there are more frequent arousals during the night and more sleep cycles during the day resulting in daytime napping. While these changes do not necessarily prevent adequate sleep time over a 24-hour period, they do lead to increased complaints of insufficient or restless sleep.

Sleep may be further disturbed by the symptoms of, for example, mus-culoskeletal and cardiorespiratory disorders. The following poor sleep habits may compound the problem: evening consumption of caffeine, alcohol, tobacco, and large meals; irregular sleep schedule, including retiring in the early evening and remaining too long in bed; insufficient exercise or physical exhaustion just before retiring; and disturbing environment (too warm, cold, light, noisy). Poor sleep habits should be changed rather than offset by medication.

Geriatric patients who get five to seven hours of sleep per day should not be prescribed hypnotics, particularly if they are not unduly fatigued during the day. As a rule, the majority of patients complaining of inability to fall asleep and/or of decreased total sleep time are found to have normal sleep for their age.

In general, the benzodiazepines are the safest and most effective anxiolytics. However, there are only a few clinical indications for their use by the elderly. They are indicated for the management of severe, disabling anxiety or panic which has resulted in significant avoidance of important activity and which prevents the patient from resolving the precipitating circumstances. They are also indicated for the treatment of specific phobias in conjunction with behavior therapy. They may also be required to treat akathisia (severe motor restlessness) induced by neuroleptics.

The benzodiazepines and their derivatives are also among the safest and most effective hypnotics. They are indicated for intractable insomnia that is unresponsive to improved sleep habits and the treatment of concurrent disorders which interfere with sleep. They may also be indicated early in a course of treatment with antidepressants. If severe insomnia and/or anxiety is a prominent and distressing symptom, a hypnotic may provide initial relief while the antidepressant is reaching therapeutic blood levels.

Adverse Effects and Contraindications

In general, the therapeutic effect of the benzodiazepines is quite brief, in the order of days or a few weeks. However, they can be remarkably effective in providing symptomatic relief with very few distressing side effects. This results in a tendency to unduly prolong their use and increase the dose or frequency of administration. The risk of physical dependency is low but that of psychological dependency is high. As a group, their most common and clinically significant adverse effect in the elderly is excessive sedation with impaired motor co-ordination.

The short-acting benzodiazepines (i.e. oxazepam, lorazepam, triazolam) result in more rebound anxiety when they are discontinued. (Rebound anxiety refers to the immediate recurrence of the symptoms for which the drug was prescribed.) In addition, when used as hypnotics, they may lead to nocturnal awakening with restlessness and anxiety.

The long-acting benzodiazepines (i.e. diazepam, flurazepam) may accu-mulate in the body over several days and result in excessive day time sedation.

All benzodiazepines may disinhibit impulsive, aggressive, and regressed behavior. Therefore, they are contraindicated as tranquillizers for patients who are prone to such behavior.

It must be noted that barbiturates are now generally regarded as absolutely contraindicated as anxiolytics and hypnotics. (They are also contraindicated for use as sedatives or tranquillizers alone or in combination with other drugs in the treatment of mental disorders.) They are subject to abuse and physical dependence and are commonly used to suicide. Physicians should not initiate treatment for anxiety or insomnia with barbiturates. For elderly patients currently prescribed barbiturates, a definitive and time limited plan for withdrawal should be made in order to terminate their prescription.

Treatment Protocol

A clinical protocol for the prescription of hypnotics is presented in Table 11.8. Short-acting benzodiazepines should be used as the initial choice of anxiolytics for geriatric patients. As in the case for other pharmacological treatments, the initial dose should be low but then increased to therapeutic levels. As an example, oxazepam should be prescribed with an initial dose of 10 mg per day. The patient's tolerance to the sedating effects can be assessed in two or three days and the dose can then be titrated upwards in 10 mg per day increments. The drug is best used in divided dosages at the times of peak symptoms during the day. The usual effective dose ranges from 10 to 40 mg per day.

TABLE 11.8

Clinical Protocol for Prescribing Hypnotic Drugs to Geriatric Patients

1. Improve sleep habits
   a. Stop daytime naps
   b. Do not consume caffeine, alcohol, tobacco or heavy meals in the evening
   c. Establish a regular sleep schedule: retire after 11:00 p.m. and arise before 8:00 a.m.
   d. Reduce noise and light and maintain average room temperature
   e. Perform physical exercise in the early evening; relaxing activity for 1 or 2 hours before retiring

2. Treat the symptoms of concurrent physical and mental disorders which disrupt sleep.

3. If necessary, a brief trial of a short-acting hypnotic in conjunction with the above-noted measures
   a. Oxazepam: 10 or 15 mg taken 1 or 2 hours before retiring
   b. Use daily for 2 to 4 nights to restore the sleep cycle and then PRN only
   c. Maximum dose: 20 daily doses per month for 3 months for chronic, intractable insomnia
   d. Discontinuation: decrease by 1 daily dose per week to avoid rebound insomnia/ anxiety

4. If a short-acting hypnotic is ineffective, a brief trial of a long-acting hypnotic
   a. Flurazepam: 15 mg taken 1 or 2 hours before retiring.
   b. Use daily for 2 to 4 nights to restore the sleep cycle and then PRN only. Assess for drug accumulation and excess daytime sedation.
   c. As above
   d. As above

Patients should be encouraged to use a full effective dose when symptoms are present but to decrease (or discontinue) the dose on those days when symptoms are minimal. *Treatment should not be continued for more than six weeks* and discontinuation should be gradual to minimize rebound anxiety. Particular attention must be paid to compliance. The effectiveness of the drugs may be prolonged by their prescription in short courses of one or two weeks which can be repeated at times of symptomatic exacerbation.

CONCLUSION

The pharmacological management of the mental disorders in the geriatric population may be very complicated. On the other hand, it may be very gratifying because many disorders are very responsive to medication alone or in combination with other measures.

Appropriate attention to prescribing principles and clinical protocols can substantially reduce the frequency of polypharmacy, non-compliance, and adverse drug reactions. While caution is warranted, pharmacological treatment must be sufficiently vigorous to ensure that patients are not deprived of effective treatment simply because of their advanced age.

REFERENCES AND SUGGESTED READINGS

Ayd F. J. 1982. "Guidelines for the Use of Lithium in the Elderly." *International Drug Therapy Newsletter.* 17: 21.

Barnes, R., R. Veith and J. Okimoto et al. 1982. "Efficacy of Antipsychotic Medications in Behaviorally Disturbed Dementia Patients." *American Journal of Psychiatry.* 139: 1170.

Berlinger W. G. and R. Spector. 1984. "Adverse Drug Reactions in the Elderly." *Geriatrics.* 39: 45.

Carlsson A. 1978. "Antipsychotic Drugs, Neurotransmitters, and Schizophrenia." *American Journal of Psychiatry.* 135: 164.

Cohen I. M., W. E. Bunney and J. O. Cole et al. 1975. "The Current Status of Lithium Therapy: Report of the APA Task Force." *American Journal of Psychiatry.* 132: 997.

Cooper A. J. and R. V. Magnus. 1984. "Strategies for the Drug Treatment of Depression." *Canadian Medical Association Journal.* 130: 383.

Cooperstock R. and J. Hill. 1982. *The Effects of Tranquillization: Benzodiazepine Use in Canada.* Health and Welfare Canada.

Gelenberg A. J. 1979. "Antidepressants in the General Hospital." *Canadian Medical Association Journal.* 120: 1377.

Greenblatt D. J., E. M. Sellers and R. I. Shader. 1982. "Drug Disposition in Old Age." *New England Journal of Medicine.* 306: 1081.

Hall M. R. P. 1973. "Drug Therapy in the Elderly." *British Medical Journal.* 4: 582.

Jefferson J. W. 1975. "A Review of the Cardiovascular Effects and Toxicity of Tricyclic Antidepressants." *Psychosomatic Medicine.* 37: 160.

Klawans H. L., C. G. Goetz and S. Perlik. 1980. "Tardive Dyskinesia: Review and Update." *American Journal of Psychiatry*. 137: 900.

Klett C. J. and E. Caffey. 1972. "Evaluating the Long-Term Need For Antiparkinson Drugs by Chronic Schizophrenics." *Archives of General Psychiatry*. 26: 374.

Lapierre Y. D., S. J. Koven and M. D. Low et al. April 23, 1985. *Report of the Expert Advisory Committee on the Short and Intermediate Acting Barbiturates*. Information Letter. Health Protection Branch. Health and Welfare Canada.

Lipowski Z. J. 1983. "Transient Cognitive Disorders (delirium, acute confusional states) in the Elderly." *American Journal of Psychiatry*. 140: 1426.

Lipsey J. R., R. G. Robinson and G. D. Pearlson et al. 1984. "Nortriptyline Treatment of Post-stroke Depression: A Double-Blind Study." *Lancet*. 297.

Martin B. A. 1986. "Electroconvulsive Therapy: Contemporary Standards of Practice." *Canadian Journal of Psychiatry*. 31:759.

Mechanic D. 1966. "Response Factors in Illness: The Study of Illness Behavior." *Social Psychiatry*. 1: 11.

Ouslander J. G. 1981. "Drug Therapy and the Elderly." *Annals of Internal Medicine*. 95: 711.

Reed K., R. C. Smith and J. C. Schoolar et al. 1980. "Cardiovascular Effects of Nortriptyline in Geriatric Patients." *American Journal of Psychiatry*. 137: 986.

Salzman C. 1982. "A Primer on Geriatric Psychopharmacology." *American Journal of Psychiatry*. 139: 67.

Schmucker D. L. 1984. "Drug Disposition in the Elderly: A Review of the Critical Factors." *Journal of the American Geriatrics Society*. 32: 144.

Task Force on the Use of Laboratory Tests in Psychiatry. 1985. "Tricyclic Antidepressants—Blood Level Measurements and Clinical Outcome: an APA Task Force Report." *American Journal of Psychiatry*. 142: 155.

Thompson T. L., M. G. Moran and A. S. Nies. 1983. "Psychotropic Drug Use in the Elderly." *New England Journal of Medicine*. 308: 194.

Varga E., A. A. Sugarman and V. Varga et al. 1982. "Prevalence of Spontaneous Oral Dyskinesia in the Elderly." *American Journal of Psychiatry*. 139: 329.

Vestel R. E. 1978. "Drug Use in the Elderly: A Review of Problems and Special Considerations." *Drugs*. 16: 358.

Vestergaard P. and M. Schou. 1985. "The Effect of Age on Lithium Dosage Requirements." *Pharmacopsychiatry*. 17: 199.

Williamson J. and J. W. Chopin. 1981. "Adverse Reactions to Prescribed Drugs in the Elderly: A Multicentre Investigation." *Age and Ageing*. 9: 73:

Zorzitto M. L. 1983. "Sleep in the Elderly." *Modern Medicine of Canada*. 38: 77.

12

Elder Abuse

Deborah M. Clark, B.S.W., C.S.W., M.Ed.

With the increase in the elderly population, especially in the over 75 age group, there has been a corresponding increase in the awareness of the complex social problems encountered by the geriatric population. Physical and emotional abuses of the elderly are included in these social problems. At present, little reliable information about the frequency of elder abuse is available due to the lack of a clear and uniform definition and also due to the under-reporting of it. In Canada, there are two sources of information regarding the frequency and distribution of the problem; a study undertaken in Manitoba (Shell 1982) and an Ontario survey of elder abuse in the community completed in 1985 by the Standing Committee on Social Development. The Manitoba study found that approximately 2.2 percent of the population aged 65 and over who were receiving care were experiencing abuse of some kind by caregivers. While the study has methodological limitations, it does offer some information regarding indicators (for example, profiles of the victims and abusers), intervention strategies, and it also emphasizes the need for more sound research to document the incidence of elder abuse. The Ontario survey also has significant methodological limitations due to a low response rate to a questionnaire. However, the tentative conclusions that may be drawn from this survey are as follows: 1) Abuse of the elderly is a problem; 2) The problem most often takes the form of neglect and/or financial abuse; 3) The physical abuse of the elderly appears to be less frequent; and, 4) The findings also indicate that the problem seems to be observed more frequently in large urban centres.

While research is limited and anecdotal, elder abuse is an issue about which health care providers to the elderly must become more aware and knowledgeable so as to make appropriate assessments and interventions.

DEFINITIONS

One of the chief difficulties in addressing elder abuse is the lack of a common working definition understood by all professionals. In the literature, definitions and types of abuse may vary among studies, thus making it exceedingly difficult to derive a comprehensive definition. Elder abuse has come to be regarded by many as anything that threatens the life or well-being of an elderly person. Definitions of abuse incorporate a wide range of phenomena, including infliction of physical pain, mental trauma, anguish and isolation, withholding basic necessities of life (for example, food, shelter, personal and medical care), and financial exploitation. The following definitions of elder abuse illustrate the difficulty in reaching consensus in this field:

1. "Abuse is any act of commission or omission which results in harm to the elderly individual and is not restricted to physical harm but rather includes financial, psychological and social abuse" (Shell 1982, 1).
2. "A continuum from simple inattention to needs to deliberate harm. It may be physical, psychological, medical or material abuse" (Johnson 1981, 32).
3. "Active intervention by caretakers such that unmet needs are created or sustained with resultant physical, psychological, or financial injury" (O'Malley 1983, 1000).
4. "Any act or behavior by a family or person providing care (formally or informally) which results in physical or mental harm or neglect of an elderly person" (Podnieks 1985, 36).

TYPES OF ABUSE

Summarizing the content of the aforementioned definitions, the following types of abuse should be included within the concept of elder abuse:

1. Physical abuse involves infliction of physical pain or discomfort through physical assault or rough handling. It may also involve sexual assault and unnecessary physical restraint.
2. Psychosocial/psychological abuse includes yelling, insulting and threatening remarks, silence, social isolation and infantilization. It may also include the violation of civil rights (for example, privacy, forced entry into an institution).
3. Financial/material abuse includes theft or misuse of money, property, or possessions.
4. Neglect involves withholding medical or personal care or failing to meet daily needs of an individual to maintain health and safety (for example, withholding nutrition, under/over medication, inadequate hygiene or inadequate supervision). Neglect may be the most prevalent form of abuse.

The elderly may be victims of any combination of the previously noted types of abuse. Mistreatment is typically a recurrent phenomena and it seems to occur more frequently to females who are frail (physically or mentally impaired), over 75 years of age, highly dependent on others for their daily needs, and living with a relative.

A profile of the abuser is as follows: a family member experiencing some form of stress (for example, financial, medical, or psychological), who is socially isolated and who may have a history of drug or alcohol abuse.

The risk factors and indicators of potential abuse to which professionals should be alert in the course of their daily work are summarized in Table 12.1. These variables are related to those addressed in the theories described below. Public health nurses and other community mental health workers are likely to come into contact with victims when the abuse is in its early stages; whereas nurses and physicians in emergency rooms may see more extreme cases (for example, physical abuse involving falls, burns, fractures, and other serious injuries).

THEORIES OF CAUSATION

At present, no single explanation for abuse of the elderly is fully satisfactory. In general terms, at least four factors have the potential to contribute to elder abuse: the health status of the individual, the caregiver's and aged relative's attitudes towards ageing, living arrangements, and finances. In addition, sudden changes in lifestyle coupled with little opportunity to escape the emotional stress of the caregiver role does little to promote satisfactory parent-child relationships. Currently, the most widely considered explanations or theories for elder abuse include the dependency of the elderly victim; the abuse as part of trans-generational violence; stressed caregivers; and, pathological caregivers.

Dependency of the Victim

These theories advance the idea that elderly persons with severe mental and physical impairments are more likely to be abused since they must rely on someone else to provide services that can be withheld or omitted for reasons beyond their control. Thus, very disabled patients with Alzheimer's disease, advanced Parkinson's disease and major strokes are at risk of inadequate care in view of their significant and often progressively increasing requirements for care. The sudden and unwanted dependency of a parent can be a source of physical, mental, as well as financial strain on family members with inadequate or maladaptive coping skills. Frequently, the burden of care falls on a middle-aged daughter caught between the competing demands of her husband, children, work, and ageing parents. A general finding of British and American studies suggests the daughter is the most likely abuser while the Manitoba study (1982) suggests the son of the victim is the most frequent abuser, followed by the daughter and then the spouse. It must also be remembered that the primary caregivers may themselves be elderly and coping with the stresses of retirement, widowhood, or physical illness while at the same time bearing responsibility for a still older dependent.

In terms of role theory, a change in the role of the elderly in relation to their adult offspring affects the way the aged parents are treated. Role reversal may be threatening to both generations and can intensify role conflicts; that is, the older person may be reluctant to relinquish authority or the adult child may have difficulty accepting increased dependency needs by a previously autonomous parent. This conflict may be the precipitant of abuse.

Trans-Generational Violence

This theory proposes that violence is a learned, normative behavior pattern in some families. According to this theory, mistreatment is potentially cyclic in nature and related to a family history of violent patterns over several generations. A life cycle approach views abuse in interactional terms with the likelihood of abused children continuing the negative behavior later in life when dependency roles are reversed.

Stressed Caregiver

This theory puts forth the view that the abuser may be influenced by a stressful environment and also may be experiencing financial difficulties, loss of employment, or chronic medical illnesses. Under these circumstances, it is very stressful for the caregiver to continue to expend time, energy and other resources in caring for the older person, particularly if the efforts are neither acknowledged nor appreciated. This frustration and uncertainty of not knowing if one's efforts are being appreciated can lead to an indifference or neglect by the caregiver. Furthermore, behavior such as combativeness, hostility, restlessness, wandering, agitation, and incontinence tend to challenge the caregiver. Retaliation may be justified in the caregiver's mind as measures to manage what may be regarded as the elderly person's uncontrollable behavior. Alternatively, some of the disturbing behavior may be viewed as purely psychological and, therefore, under the person's conscious control. Thus, for example, deliberate incontinence may be seen as deserving punishment.

Pathological Caregiver

This theory contends that abusers have personality traits or character disorders that cause them to be abusive. A number of investigators note the history of drug or alcohol abuse in the caregiver. Included in the category of the pathological caregiver are mentally retarded or adult children with schizophrenia who may be unable to provide proper care or make appropriate judgments. In these cases, the actual care needs of the aged individual may be minimal but due to the inherent emotional problems in the abuser, the elderly person becomes a victim of mistreatment. The abusing caregiver may have had a past history of abuse occurring in childhood—whether actual or perceived.

ASSESSMENT

In order to assess for elder abuse, the professional must develop an index of suspicion. Observation of the following factors should alert the professional to the possibility of elder abuse: frail elderly females who are highly dependent on others for their daily care; history of an older person suffering repeated injuries with contradictory explanations offered by the caregiver; and the presence of malnutrition, dehydration, or medication abuse in an older person. A more complete outline of the risk factors associated with potential abuse situations is provided in Table 12.1. Knowledge of abuse dynamics combined with interviewing skills to establish positive relationships with older individuals and caregivers are required in order to obtain the necessary information about sensitive subject matters. In the initial assessment, several issues must be addressed. Is the elderly person in immediate danger of physical injury? If not, and if immediate separation is not indicated, is s/he mentally competent to make decisions affecting her/his future? What is the degree and significance of impairment of the individual? What community services might help to meet the individual's needs? What is the level of the family involvement in meeting the elderly person's needs or in contributing to the abusive situation? Are the older person and family willing to accept outside interventions?

TABLE 12.1

Risk Factors for Potential Abuse of the Elderly

1. **Profile of the potential victim**
   a. Female over 75 years of age
   b. Severely disabled by chronic and/or progressive disease (for example, Alzheimer's disease, Parkinson's disease, stroke, mental illness)
   c. Living with a relative who is the primary or sole caregiver
   d. History of recurring or unexplained injuries
   e. Showing signs of malnutrition, dehydration, poor hygiene, or drug toxicity
   f. Socially isolated

2. **Profile of the potential abuser**
   a. Relationship to the potential victim: daughter, son, or spouse
   b. Sudden onset of unwanted dependency with forced assumption of the caregiver role. Resents role reversal with parent
   c. Financial stress resulting from caregiving
   d. History of drug or alcohol abuse
   e. History of severe mental disorder (for example, schizophrenia) or mental retardation
   f. Family history of violence, particularly of being physically or sexually abused
   g. Mention of punishment by the older person or caregiver
   h. Social isolation of the caregiver
   i. Refusal of community or medical services
   j. Caregiver is hostile, irritable, or suspicious when questioned
   k. Demonstrates poor impulse control

Silence and denial on the part of the elderly make detection and assessment of abuse difficult. Abused elderly persons may believe that either little can be done or they may fear threats of retaliation, abandonment, or placement. Thus, they may not co-operate with the professional. The alternative to abuse and neglect may be perceived as more frightening than the current situation. The elderly rarely (or with great difficulty) report incidents of abuse committed by family members upon whom they depend. Instead, the abused may complain of depression, anxiety, or fear. It is important to note that the caregiver and the elderly person may minimize the seriousness of the abuse. The ageing parent may want to avoid the shame and humiliation of admitting s/he raised an abusing son/daughter.

In addition to the variables noted in Table 12.1, some observations about the caregiver should raise the index of suspicion of the possibility of abuse. These observations include the following: the caregiver demonstrates loss of control or fear of losing control; gives a contradictory history; is unable to explain an injury; demands unusual treatment for a minor problem; or, underreacts to a serious problem and refuses consent for diagnostic studies.

The parent's manner and, more importantly, the nature and quality of the parent/child interaction should be noted. Is the parent unduly afraid or agitated in the presence of the adult child or perhaps overly quiet and passive? Is the adult child passive or withdrawn (a lack of response may suggest disinterest in care issues and recommended resources)? It is essential to locate the primary caregiver and assess his or her social, emotional state, drug or alcohol history, and concern regarding control issues. In cases that appear to indicate neglect, it is important to assess the caregiver's level of understanding, knowledge of available resources and the elder's willingness to accept care.

In terms of assessing the older individual in the home, it is recommended that initially the patient and the caregiver be interviewed separately, followed by a joint interview. It is important to follow a line of inquiry from general non-threatening questions to more direct, emotionally-laden issues in a calm, unhurried manner, providing reassurance as needed. An important skill in interviewing the abusing caregiver is to avoid introducing further provocation that may have consequences for the aged parent. This may require subsequent interviews and the ability to recognize when to terminate an interview before it goes out of control. It is also necessary that the professional be non-judgmental. Premature assumptions regarding the older person's mental status (for example, demented, paranoid) should be avoided. A thorough assessment necessitates being observant for evidence of trauma, burns, poor nutritional status, and any recent deterioration in general functioning, both physical and mental. It may also be useful to inquire into the typical day of the older person/caregiver. It is worthwhile to inquire into the adult child's perception of past parenting roles.

In abuse cases, the line of inquiry involves a series of questions which must be answered in order to decide appropriate management for the elderly person who has been abused in the home. Basic to the overall inquiry is learning if the abused person wants to remain in the home. If the answer is yes, can the individual's care needs be adequately met by family and outside service providers? Also, are the older person and family willing to accept outside intervention? If answers to both these questions are in the affirmative then the health professional should make appropriate referrals to community services for counselling, nursing and homemaking services, day programs, respite care, and caregiver support groups. In cases where the older person's care needs cannot be adequately met by a combination of informal and formal support services, then the family must decide if they are willing to accept inadequate care to maintain the elderly relative at home.

Professionals may encounter situations where the abused elderly person does not want to remain in the home setting. If after a thorough assessment, the professional finds that leaving the home is in the best interest of the older person, then counselling efforts should be directed to exploring alternate living arrangements, that is, a seniors' apartment, a residential care facility, or a nursing home. In the event that the individual's reasons are unjustified, then the professional's role is to provide family counselling with a view to exploring all available options, (for example, temporary placement, day programming).

INTERVENTION

There is no single formula regarding intervention. It is likely that several factors are involved in any given case of elder abuse and that it will require several levels of intervention as well as the development of new helping skills. In addition, the issue of intra-family violence must be seen in a broad societal context of an increased tolerance for violence. If professionals are to intervene appropriately and effectively they need to be aware and knowledgeable of the following: 1) profile of the abused (the demographic and sociologic information); 2) the theories of causation to assess and understand causal factors; 3) the available community resources; 4) a knowledge of the normal ageing process; and, 5) a knowledge of self regarding attitudes towards violence, ageing, and dependency.

In order to intervene and prevent cases of geriatric abuse within the family, two major obstacles must be overcome. First, professionals may deny that the problem exists and that its frequency may be increasing. Second, there is a lack of procedures for case detection.

Prevention by Reducing Risk Factors

The initial objective of intervention strategies is to reduce risk factors for abuse. This is possible only in the broadest sense of increasing the early recognition of abuse and its risk factors. There is a need to increase public awareness of the problem of elder abuse and to increase professional knowledge and skill regarding the assessment of possible and potential abuse. Middle-aged families need education and guidance regarding normal ageing and the needs of the elderly. Clearly, professional training needs to be augmented in order to recognize the dynamics of abuse and to initiate prompt treatment. The ideal strategy is to deal with the problem before rather than after the abuse occurs. The development of multidisciplinary elder abuse teams is an effective way to provide ongoing consultation and education for other professionals.

Professionals should take an advocacy position to represent the views and special needs of the elderly. Myths and stereotypes regarding the aged must be challenged in order to effect changes in those attitudes which result in the mistreatment of the elderly in society at all levels. Professionals are in a position to identify gaps in the service delivery system to the elderly and to work to develop and co-ordinate support services needed by those who are abused.

Research is needed to increase knowledge of geriatric abuse in both the family and institutional settings and to develop a screening assessment instrument for community workers.

Early Detection and Management

This involves the early detection of abuse and securing appropriate medical and nursing care. Access and intervention has to be negotiated with both the individual and the caregiver. Professionals must be aware of and knowledgeable about community resources in order to help increase the family's ability to cope with the 24-hour care demands of a physically and/or mentally impaired older adult. Services such as home help agencies, legal and financial aid, "Meals-On-Wheels", visiting nurses, transportation, emergency shelter, medical and mental health services are all important resources. Instruction in self-care to reduce the dependency of the older individual is needed as well. The intervention plan must take into account the structure and function of the family system and this can be best assessed through multiple interviews and observations.

Counselling is essential to those families assuming the care of an ageing relative. The focus of counselling should be to assess the caregiver's functional capacities, to identify role conflicts, to clarify expectations, and to strengthen the family's overall ability to cope. All family members involved in caregiving need to receive information regarding normal ageing and ways to extend the caregiving circle. (For example, volunteers, friends, neighbors and peers can be enlisted as additional service providers so the dependency needs can be shared.)

Families may benefit from many specific types of counselling under various circumstances. Counselling may need to be available in the form of crisis intervention and/or ongoing family therapy. Long term follow-up should be available and not viewed as failure. The caregiver needs to receive support in his or her role and referral to appropriate self-help groups can be effective. Concrete assistance and advice in caring for the physically and/or mentally impaired elderly in the home is essential, (for example, advice about home safety, medications, environmental modifications). There are cases which may require immediate intervention by professionals. These include situations when the caregiver is too incapacitated; when the potential for severe injury to the patient cannot be adequately reduced by the caregiver; or, when essential medical or psychiatric care is required.

Prevention of Further Abuse

The final level of care has, as its goal, reducing the effects of abuse and may involve respite care and at times temporary or permanent placement. Ongoing individual and family counselling may be further strategies utilized by the professional. Generally, intervention should promote the least restrictive alternative to ongoing abuse while respecting the rights to privacy and self-determination. While caregivers may be contributing to abuse, the family unit is potentially the most nurturing environment for the elderly person.

CONCLUSION

In conclusion, professionals need to direct further efforts towards changing negative attitudes towards the elderly. Ageism is a form of prejudice which can have deleterious effects on the health and psychological well-being of the elderly. While treatment efforts of professionals should be directed to maintaining people in their homes where possible and practical, the possibility for physical and emotional abuse must be recognized. Further research is required to document the frequency of geriatric abuse. In this regard, an acceptable definition of what constitutes elder abuse would be helpful. Finally, a review of intervention strategies and outcomes should be conducted to improve the community response to this complex problem.

An unfortunate last resort may be the development of legal remedies (for example, mandatory reporting analogous to child abuse). This may be required if efforts by health care professionals are unsuccessful in identifying cases. All this must be considered in the context of maintaining a balance between protecting the individual versus preservation of individual rights. Professionals must avoid taking a paternalistic attitude toward the elderly which may override the individual's right to self-determination and privacy.

REFERENCES AND SUGGESTED READINGS

Anderson C. February 1981. "Abuse and Neglect Among the Elderly." *Journal of Gerontological Nursing.* 7: 77.

Anderson L. and M. Thobaden. December 1984. "Clients in Crisis." *American Journal of Gerontological Nursing.* 10: 6.

Beck C. and D. Ferguson. June 1981. "Aged Abuse." *Gerontological Nursing.* 7: 333.

Bookin D. and R. Dunkle. January 1985. "Elder Abuse: Issues for the Practitioner." *Social Casework.* 66: 3.

Falcioni D. April 1982. "Assessing the Abused Elderly." *Journal of Gerontological Nursing.* 8: 208.

Ferguson D. and C. Beck. October 1983. "HALF—A Tool to Assess Elder Abuse Within the Family." *Geriatric Nursing.* 4: 301.

Fulmer T., S. Street and K. Carr. May/June 1984. "Abuse of Elderly: Screening and Detection." *Journal of Emergency Nursing.* 10: 131.

Ghent W., N. DaSylva and M. Farren. March 1985. "Family Violence: Guidelines for Recognition and Management." *Canadian Medical Association Journal.* 132: 541.

Giordano N.H. and J. Giordano. May/June 1984. "Elder Abuse: Review of the Literature." *Social Work.* 29: 232.

Johnson D. January/February 1981. "Abuse of the Elderly." *Nurse Practitioner.* 6: 29.

O'Malley T.A., D.E. Everitt, H.C. O'Malley and E.W. Campion. 1983. "Identifying and Preventing Family-Mediated Abuse and Neglect of Elderly Persons." *Annals of Internal Medicine.* 98: 998.

Podnieks E. December 1985. "Elder Abuse: It's Time We Did Something About It." *Canadian Nurse.* 81: 36.

Rathbone-McCuan E. May 1980. "Elderly Victims of Family Violence and Neglect." *Social Casework*. 61: 296.

Rathbone-McCuan E. and B. Voyles. February 1982. "Case Detection of Abused Elderly Parents." *American Journal of Psychiatry*. 139: 189.

Shell D.J. 1982. *Protection of the Elderly: A Study of Elder Abuse*. Winnipeg Manitoba Association on Gerontology.

Standing Committee on Social Development. 1985. *Report of Survey of Elder Abuse in the Community*. Toronto: The Committee.

Part Four
FAMILY AND COMMUNITY RESOURCES

13

Family Supports

Deborah M. Clark, B.S.W., C.S.W., M.Ed. and
E. Anne Lennox, R.N., B.Sc.N., M.P.H

This chapter describes the professional's role in supporting families who are caring for elderly relatives. Background information including a demographic description of the ageing Canadian population is presented. An overview of the family life cycle and basic needs of caregivers are also explored. The final section examines institutional placement and the crisis it creates for families.

Families are experiencing a variety of problems and strains as a result of social change. The contemporary family may be overwhelmed with the responsibilities of child rearing, career demands, and the changing roles of men and women. At the same time, the expectations for families to perform caring and nurturing roles for their elderly relatives has not diminished. In contrast to the common misperception, it is known that a great proportion of the elderly are neither isolated from their families nor abandoned by them in institutions. Empirical studies have demonstrated that the modal family of present day North America is still an extended family in which the elderly, although they may live in separate households, remain active participants in the primary kin network. Further, the majority of the elderly live either in the same household or within ten minutes of one of their children, and up to 70 to 80 percent of elderly persons have personal contact with at least one of their children in any given week.

The presence of an older person requiring care is frequently a source of stress on the family, particularly on the primary caregiver. Anxiety, guilt, fatigue, physical illness, restricted social contacts, and depression are often the hallmarks of an adult caring for an elderly relative. It is crucial to develop ways to mitigate the stress of caregiving families in order to support them in their vital role.

The concept of burden is synonymous with the effects of caregiving. Objective measures of burden have been investigated such as the impact of caregiving on family relationships, social activities, health of the caregiver, and employment changes. Equally important in determining burden is the caregiver's unique experience of the situation. Consideration of both these factors will improve the quality of care professionals provide to families. The frail elderly, caregivers, and families represent an extremely heterogeneous group of individuals with marked variation in personality, life experience, and family functioning. The problem-solving skills of caregivers and their ability to ask for and accept support from formal and informal sources also vary. Factors such as cultural differences, education, gender, age, and socio-economic status are examples of variables which influence caregiving.

Of the approximately 2.5 million Canadians 65 years and over (representing 10 percent of the total population), approximately 90 percent are living in the community with the remainder in institutions. The rate of institutionalization increases with age. For example, one tenth of the population 65 to 80 years of age is institutionalized compared to one fourth of the population more than 80 years of age. Part of the reason for this is that the incidence of mental and physical frailty increase with age. Institutionalization is usually the last resort for families and occurs when the burden for the caregiver becomes too great. Hence, the support provided to families by professional caregivers is an integral component of community care.

DEFINITIONS

Before proceeding, some clarification of the terminology in this chapter may be of benefit. Reference to a "primary caregiver" is in recognition of the fact that there is typically one individual within the family who assumes the primary caregiving function. Traditionally, this person is a middle-aged daughter or daughter-in-law. It is likely more acceptable to an aged parent to allow one family member to provide personal care rather than a variety of family members and/or outside service providers. This form of caregiving will be referred to as part of the informal support system.

Individuals working with the elderly and their families are referred to as "professional helpers". This group of professionals comprises the formal support system and includes aides, homemakers, nurses, occupational therapists, physicians, psychologists, social workers, and speech therapists. No one discipline has all the skills or expertise to address the many problems encountered in working with the elderly. It is only through a multi-disciplinary team approach that co-ordinated care is feasible.

A "support system" involves one or more individuals with whom another is connected in an emotional relationship and who may be relied upon for assistance. The first experience of a support system is within the family which protects and nurtures the development of the next generation. The elderly person may have a support system which includes family, friends, neighbors or a concerned landlord. These are referred to as "informal supports" in that they develop spontaneously, either from a previously close emotional relationship or through a basic concern for the individual. This informal support system may be instrumental in maintaining the elderly in the community through help with personal care or supervision, shopping, transportation, arranging social services, or providing emotional support. "Formal support services" are those that have been arranged through a social/health agency, such as a family service agency or home care program. The individual has to meet program eligibility criteria in order to receive service.

It is generally accepted that elders and their families prefer home care to institutionalization and, further, that professional helpers should explore and utilize all support services to that end. Nevertheless, it must also be acknowledged that a small segment of the older population has daily care needs that are well beyond what family and/or formal support services can adequately provide. In these cases of advanced mental and/or physical frailty, institutionalization may be the most feasible plan of care. Later in this chapter, the problems encountered by elderly persons and families facing the prospect of institutional placement are described.

THE FAMILY LIFE CYCLE

A family has a life cycle of its own and, over the course of years undergoes many changes. The family may be conceptualized as passing through several phases: pre-parental, parental, post-parental, and ageing. In the pre-parental phase, a newly married couple is involved in working through several tasks; leaving the families of origin, establishing the marital relationship, and maintaining a joint household. A couple in the parental phase assumes responsibilities of child rearing and building family relationships. The post-parental phase occurs when the children are grown and have left home. Without the children between them, the couple may be faced with redefining their relationship. The developmental tasks of this phase may also include resolution of earlier conflicts with parents. This involves adult children accepting parents as they are and becoming a dependable source of support to them. The ageing phase may involve taking on grandparenting roles as well as coping with retirement and the transition to activities other than those related to employment.

Throughout these phases, the family structure is a dynamic entity; that is, the parent/child relationship continues to be negotiated and renegotiated throughout the entire life span of both generations. The direction of support often changes in the later stages of the family life cycle—from parents to children, to that of adult children to elderly parents. The social and physical dependency resulting from advancing age may contribute to changes over time in the power and authority structure of a family. This redistribution of power within the family may lead to struggle and conflict among family members. Nevertheless, families must be prepared to adjust roles in response to an ageing relative's increasing frailty. Psychological factors such as denial of ageing may hinder the family's ability to make this adaptation to the caregiving role. Financial strain and job pressures may further drain the family's resources to cope with the impact of the ageing relative.

THE NEEDS OF CAREGIVERS

Caregivers have five primary needs: emotional support, education, support groups, information on community resources, and relief from the caregiving role when the burden becomes onerous. Each of these identified needs will be examined in relation to caregivers and the role of professional helpers.

Emotional Support

Emotional support can be defined as affection, feeling wanted and cared for, as well as specific support during a crisis. Caregivers may obtain emotional support from the informal support system which has been described earlier and which includes family, friends, and neighbors. In general, the burden of care is found to be less when supports are readily available, such as, frequent visitors to the household. This observation substantiates one aspect of caregivers' needs for emotional support which may be fulfilled by family relationships or friends.

Caregivers may be referred to professional helpers such as visiting nurses, occupational therapists, or social workers in order to obtain emotional support. It is the professional helper's job to assess the existing individual and family resources, and to help the caregiver mobilize more support as needed. There may be a number of reasons why caregivers have difficulty obtaining necessary emotional support. It should be noted that caregivers may be reluctant or embarrassed to share problems with others for fear of being seen as complaintive or disloyal to their relative. For others, there may be a social stigma attached to requesting or accepting outside help. Others reject help offered to them because of difficulty relinquishing control to formal support services. A caregiver may feel that no one outside the family system can provide a comparable quality of care. Past rivalries within the family may also complicate the utilization of formal support services. Outside help may be more acceptable to families when emphasis is placed on the need to maintain personal health in order to continue caregiving.

The caregiver may look to professional helpers for "permission" to ask another family member to take over temporarily, in order to have a complete break from the caregiving role. Caregivers may need help to understand the complexity of emotions that are a part of the experience. Frustration, guilt, ambivalence, hostility, and depression are recognized emotional reactions to the strain of caregiving. Emotional support, whether from informal or formal sources, is essential to sustain the caregiver's role.

Education

The purpose of education is to improve the quality of care to the relative while minimizing the burden to the caregiver. Gaining an intellectual under-standing of the situation will facilitate emotional acceptance of this stressful life event. Healthy coping is promoted by specific education for caregivers. Topics which should be included in an educational program are the process of normal ageing, information on specific illnesses, medications, special care procedures, and management strategies. Community resources and alternatives to community care should also be included.

In those instances involving chronic and progressive disorders, caregivers need specific information about the medical diagnosis, the cause of the illness, and the prognosis for the person for whom they are responsible. Families frequently have sketchy information or none at all. They may not have sought an explanation from the family doctor nor insisted upon medical investigations to determine the cause of disability. Families may be given dismissive information about functional losses. For example, a statement such as, "Your mother's getting old. What do you expect at her age?", conveys an attitude which precludes full clinical investigation and treatment. Families need specific guidelines to negotiate the medical system to ensure that an adequate medical work-up is obtained. The professional helper's role may involve referral to physicians who have both the expertise and the interest in treating the elderly. Educating caregivers about the normal ageing process may help them seek appropriate medical care when required.

Caregivers sometimes believe that medications cure or arrest the underlying disease process. As a result, families may at some point demand multiple consultations in the hope of finding a miracle cure. Families may also need assistance in modifying expectations of their relatives and in making necessary environmental adjustments in order to maintain them at home.

In addition to the factual information needed, families require education to identify and understand the emotional reactions to chronic illness. Because of the intense emotional bond that may have existed prior to initiation of the caregiving situation, interpreting behavior and personality changes to the caregiver is very important and usually requires considerable tact. This is particularly so for families caring for a dementing relative where behavior problems may be extremely distressing aspects of the disease. For example, behavior such as aggression, wandering, swearing or emotional outbursts may escalate the caregiver's feelings of burden. (See also Chapter 10.) Organizations, such as the Parkinson's Foundation, Stroke Recovery, or the Alzheimer's Society provide practical behavior management strategies which are available in printed form.

Discussion of the cause of a disorder like dementia may require the caregiver to face reality—not only will the relative not improve, but a time may come when caregiving at home is no longer feasible. Acceptance of the need for placement may represent a major dilemma for the caregiver, requiring an extended period of time for its resolution. The realization that in times of crisis backup help may well be unavailable can cause a tremendous amount of anxiety and resentment in the caregiver. Therefore, one of the professional helper's responsibilities is to actively explore future care planning and placement with the caregiver. This is a vital educational service because it may substantively decrease fears of feeling trapped with no hope of escaping the burden of the caregiver role.

Support Groups

Support groups provide opportunities for caregivers to vent emotions, receive education, and share information with others. A caregiver support group creates a temporary community of people who can discuss particular home situations, describe attempts at problem-solving, and express unresolved feelings. This opportunity to give and receive support may also help the caregiver articulate needs more clearly. Participants may experience great relief to know their emotional experiences are normal and shared by others. Group members may meet more experienced caregivers who have lived with similar problems or worse, for even longer periods. Group membership may foster a sense of competency and self-confidence for caregivers. An exchange of ideas can take place in the caregiver's support group as the unique situations are discussed. Peer confrontation can occur with members challenging each other to take action. Hence, a support group can be a place where a participant can introduce a problematic situation, ask for assistance, and become the focus of the group's problem-solving energy. A support group may be a potent means of promoting personal growth and providing information and emotional support to caregivers.

The professional helper can play a variety of roles in the initiation and maintenance of caregiver support groups. These roles include the following: identifying and referring potential group members; acting as group facilitator; or providing consultative services on request. In working with families, professionals may identify and establish groups for caregivers with special needs which are not directly addressed by existing support groups. Multicultural differences, the need for respite care, or for a specific disease-related support group are examples of unmet needs of caregivers.

Community Resources

Professional referrals to community resources such as home care, respite care, day programs, and family support groups can be an essential service to caregiving families.

Families require someone to act as a referral agent to other services and to co-ordinate the care they need. Professional helpers must be knowledgeable about community resources so as to offer appropriate referral information. They should also be prepared to act as case managers to minimize duplication and fragmentation of formal support services. As a case manager, one designated professional should remain involved as long as the family requires assistance. It must be remembered that needs change over time. Therefore, it may not be satisfactory to put services in place and then abandon the contact. Even when services are available, families may need help to gain access to them. Updating knowledge on community resources and linking families to relevant services is basic to community care of the elderly. (For further information see Chapter 15.)

Respite Care

Respite care should be an essential part of the spectrum of services available to caregivers. The majority of caregivers want to continue their role for as long as they are able to do so. Respite care involves the provision of temporary services so that caregivers may have psychological and physical relief from the burden of care at home. Though the activities involved in providing respite are directed to the elderly person, the primary beneficiary is the caregiver who receives relief, for a few hours to a few weeks, from regular caregiving tasks.

Respite programs may differ in format, depending upon location. The following are some examples of different respite programs:

1. Where the elderly person lives: A respite worker (paid or volunteer) may come to the person's residence for a scheduled block of time.
2. In the respite worker's home: The elderly person is left for a period of time. This is similar to foster care, but is a short-term stay rather than an extended living arrangement.
3. In a group program setting: An elderly person may be brought to a seniors' centre or a day-care centre in order to participate in a structured program.
4. In a home for the aged or nursing home: This is an arrangement for stays of 24 hours or longer, up to several weeks.

While respite care is not widely available, it is incumbent upon professionals to inform families of relief services where they exist. Community professionals are in a key position to advocate for increased government funding of respite care services.

INSTITUTIONAL PLACEMENT

Families respond in many ways when a marked change occurs in an elderly relative's mental and/or physical functioning. Some caregivers deny a relative's disabilities and, therefore, make no realistic plan to provide support. Other caregivers recognize disabilities and seek the aid of community support services, yet still have difficulty handling personal reactions to the relative's losses. Immediate placement may be the first course of action for some who feel threatened by the relative's deterioration. Arranging support services and/or placement may occur when families are in the midst of anticipatory grief. The source of this grief is the caregiver's realization of the relative's declining health and change in status, that is, a move from autonomy to a level of dependency. The relative's imminent death may precipitate anxiety in the caregiver. This anxiety relates to a heightened awareness of personal mortality. Families who have long standing difficulties communicating are likely to have increased problems when stressed with the elderly relative's deterioration and the need to make decisions about institutional care.

There is no simple means of predicting the point at which placement may be necessary for an elderly relative. In general, the elderly with families tend to enter institutions at a later age than those with no available family support. The placement decision is complex and overshadowed by emotions, family values, and outside pressures. Placement may be precipitated by a number of factors: deterioration in the physical or mental status, when reciprocation in an emotional relationship is no longer possible, or when the caregiver has no relief from the situation.

At the time of placement, families may experience a mixture of anxiety, intense guilt and relief along with nagging doubts about whether or not they are doing the best thing for all concerned. Therefore, preparation of both the older person and the family for admission to long-term care is advisable. Selection of an appropriate facility is dependent upon a thorough assessment of the individual to determine the level of nursing care required. Clinical experience suggests that those older people who have preparation for a move to an institution fare better than those who are admitted with little or no preparation. It is helpful for both caregivers and the elderly to actually visit the institution beforehand to familiarize themselves with the surroundings.

During the admission process, caregivers may benefit from counselling to accept the expressed resentment of the older person who may feel abandoned. Resolution of any crisis that occurs at the time of institutionalization may be facilitated by a number of factors, such as, the institution's policies that promote the older person's autonomy and interaction with family; the family's ability to make appropriate use of the services available; and the unique personality of the older person entering the institution.

Established family patterns of interaction need not be broken once placement occurs. Caring professional staff members and responsive administrative policies promote continued family involvement in the first few weeks after admission. Attention to these environmental influences may also reduce the older person's sense of abandonment. Staff and family should be close allies to ensure optimal care of the elderly relative. Provision of information regarding the new resident's likes/dislikes, personality, and abilities/disabilities, may ease the adjustment into the institution. At the same time, the primary caregiver may feel the need to have a vital role in the older person's care. A care facility's commitment to fostering family ties is conveyed by such things as open visiting hours, sponsorship of family nights, encouragement of the older person to attend family events, and allowing families to assist with personal care.

New concerns and issues may confront caregivers after a relative's admission to a long-term care facility. In some situations, family relationships deteriorate and there is an emotional and/or physical withdrawal. The progressive deterioration of the relative's condition may precipitate a need for a more intensive level of nursing care. This crisis again forces the family to confront the very real issue of the mortality of the relative. Caregivers may need the services of a professional helper to work through their own anticipatory grief in order to continue the supportive role. Families may need counselling to visit relatives and, when it becomes too difficult, permission to visit less frequently.

CONCLUSION

Throughout this chapter, the significant role of families in the provision of social and health care services to elderly relatives has been emphasized. There is no question that it is the level of caregiving by the family that is most instrumental in delaying or preventing institutionalization of the elderly. While the role of support to caregiving families has been stressed, it is not yet clear to what extent social support mediates the stress of caregiving. Thus, further research is necessary to understand the long-term effects of social support as well as to identify those caregivers who are most likely to benefit from support.

There are significant gaps in formal support services to caregiving families. Most prominent among these is the lack of available and accessible respite care. Families maintain the struggle to care for frail elderly relatives while offers of community support services by professionals are frequently too little and too late. A professional helper's role should include the identification of gaps in service and the development of a network of service providers to advocate for the creation of special needs programs. Timely and full assessment plus the provision of assistance at critical intervals must be provided. Otherwise, caregivers become physically and emotionally overwhelmed and frustrated from the lack of help and interest in their plight.

REFERENCES AND SUGGESTED READINGS

Blenkner M. 1965. "Social Work and Family Relationships in Later Life With Some Thoughts on Filial Maturity." *Social Structure and the Family*. Ed. E. Shanas and G. Streib. Englewood Cliffs: Prentice Hall.

Chappell N. L., L. A. Strain and A. A. Blackford. 1986. *Aging and Health Care: A Special Perspective*. Toronto: Holt, Rinehart and Winston.

Clark N. and W. Rakowski. 1983. "Family Caregivers of Older Adults: Improving Helping Skills." *Gerontologist*. 23: 637.

Lidoff L. 1983. *Respite Companion Program Model*. Washington: The National Council on the Aging, Inc.

Morycz R. K. 1980. "An Exploration of Senile Dementia and Family Burden." *Clinical Social Work Journal*. 8: 16.

Poulshock S. W. October 1982. *The Effects on Families of Caring For Impaired Elderly in Residence*. Cleveland.

Poulshock S. W. and G. T. Deimling. 1984. "Families Caring for Elders in Residence: Issues in the Measurement of Burden." *Journal of Gerontology*. 39: 230.

Reece D. and T. Walz. Spring 1983. "Intergenerational Care Providers of Non-institutionalized Frail Elderly: Characteristics and Consequences." *Journal of Gerontological Social Work*. 5: 21.

Shanas E. August 1973. "Family—Kin Networks in Cross-cultural Perspective." *Journal of Marriage and the Family*. 35: 505.

Solomon R. 1983. "Serving Families of the Institutionalized Aged: The Four Crises." *Journal of Gerontological Social Work*. 5: 83.

Statistics Canada. June 1984. *Census*. Catalogue #91-210. Ottawa: Government of Canada.

Sussman M. B. 1959. "The Isolated Nuclear Family: Fact or Fiction." *Social Problems*. 6: 333.

Verwoerdt A. 1981. *Clinical Geropsychiatry*. 2nd ed. Baltimore: Williams and Wilkins.

Zarit S., K. Reever and J. Bach-Peterson. 1980. "Relatives of the Impaired Elderly: Correlates of Feelings of Burden." *Gerontologist*. 20: 649.

Respite Care for the Frail Elderly. 1983. Albany: Centre for the Study of Aging, Inc.

14

Community Resources

Lynda A. Perry, M.S.W., C.S.W.

Effective use of the wide variety of services existing in any community is the key to maintaining frail elderly people in their own home environment and at their optimum level of functioning. It is the responsibility of all health care professionals working with the elderly to be thoroughly aware of available services or, alternatively, to arrange consultation with or referral to another professional who is knowledgeable. In keeping with this responsibility, it is essential to consider the older client/patient as a whole person whose unmet needs may well extend beyond the scope of the skills and expertise that can be provided by any single discipline, agency, or individual practitioner.

ACQUIRING KNOWLEDGE ABOUT COMMUNITY RESOURCES

To use resources effectively for the benefit of clients, it is important to know not only what services exist and their eligibility criteria, but also the nuances in the way the agency provides services, the actual type of client in which the program is most interested, and the way the stated eligibility criteria are interpreted by the program staff. For example, in Ontario, in order to receive government funding for care in a nursing home, an individual must have a doctor complete a multiple-choice functional assessment. Often people, particularly the demented, are declared ineligible for assistance simply because the physician does not understand the nuances of the assessment form. The physician may state that the patient is able to go to the dining room unassisted because s/he is capable of walking. However, this limited assessment of this particular function does not take into consideration the assistance involved in repeatedly reminding the patient that it is meal time and in directing or accompanying the patient to be sure s/he does not get lost.

Similarly, many programs require that the client have identifiable goals which can be expected to be achieved in a specified time period. Often people are denied admission to such programs because the person making the referral describes them as needing long-term maintenance only. With a little creative thinking, however, it is usually possible to establish an achievable short-term goal which will facilitate admission to the program. If necessary, involvement with the program may be extended through a series of short-term goals or alternative services can be planned when the person is discharged from a short-term program.

Developing personal contacts within key resources is often useful to ease communication and to facilitate the acceptance of clients into programs. It is also important to develop a reputation for referring suitable clients and for being honest about the strengths and weaknesses of clients. The development of a history of favorable contacts with an agency becomes most important in negotiating the acceptance of a client who does not clearly meet the eligibility requirements of the program. A certain flexibility may be possible with frank discussion of the particular circumstances.

Acquiring comprehensive knowledge of community resources is not a simple matter for a number of reasons. In large metropolitan areas, the complexity of the service delivery system may be overwhelming. When services to seniors are offered by small neighborhood based agencies or by those with strict catchment boundaries, it is not unusual to find that the service which was so useful to one client is not available to a neighbor on the next street. In small rural communities, the number and diversity of formal services may be quite limited and it may be more important to know how to gain access to informal supports such as neighbors and service clubs.

To find out about resources within a community a first step is to consult directories which may be available from information services or local co-ordinating bodies. Participation on inter-agency committees is a good way to learn about other agencies and to develop personal contacts. An information service should be consulted whenever a client is seen who could benefit from a service which is not available. This helps establish data to verify gaps in service or to identify an existing service which can meet the client's need. Accompanying clients on a first visit to a program, arranging for a personal tour, and attending open houses are all ways of increasing awareness of a particular agency.

ASSESSING THE CLIENT

In order to make an effective referral to a program or agency, it is necessary to know the client well since a good referral may be able to meet more than one of a client's needs. For example, a client found to be malnourished may admit that s/he has not been eating properly. A wide range of services might be considered to address this problem. These services include psychiatric treatment, help with shopping, "meals-on-wheels", a diner's club, a homemaker, or admission to a nursing home. In order to decide which service may be most appropriate, a more complete assessment is required. That assessment must address a number of specific questions.

1. Is the client depressed? Anorexia, profound weight loss or malnutrition may be a symptom of severe depression. Therefore, the client should be assessed for other symptoms of this mental disorder as described in Chapter 9.

2. Has the client forgotten how to obtain groceries or how to cook? Impaired memory, disorientation and dyspraxia are symptoms of dementia which may interfere with activities of daily living such as food preparation. Therefore, the client should be assessed for the specific symptoms of dementia as described in Chapter 9.

3. Are other activities of daily living impaired? Difficulty managing finances and dressing appropriately would be further indications of possible dementia. The ability to calculate and to co-ordinate movements may also be impaired in dementia. Neglect of cleaning and home maintanence may be an indication of a drinking problem which is interfering with eating. (See also Chapter 8.)

4. Can any recent precipitant of a change in behavior be identified? A large number of events may contribute to or precipitate a deterioration in the health or behavior of an elderly person at home. Such events may include a change in the availability of support (e.g. a neighbor away on holiday), an emotional loss (e.g. a death in the family), concurrent physical illness, and inclement weather. The assessment should include some probing questions about recent changes in circumstances.

5. What does the client think may be helpful under the circumstances? It is important to determine the client's insight into the presence of a problem and the need for assistance. It is also important to respect personal preferences.

LINKING THE CLIENT WITH THE SERVICE

For some clients, simply giving the information that a service exists and perhaps the telephone number is all that is needed to link the client to the service. However, for most clients, more direct support is required. Often it is necessary to spend a great deal of time discussing the client's needs and possible ways that specific services could help. It is important to listen for any resistance to accepting help and to understand and deal with any concerns that are voiced or implied. Working through such resistance involves more than reassuring the client. Underlying concerns and past experiences must be taken seriously and acknowledged before the client will be able to consider accepting the referral. For example, a client may be reluctant to allow a public health nurse to visit because s/he associates public health with maintenance of hygiene standards. S/he is insulted at the suggestion and fears the neighbors would stigmatize her/him. Information about the range of services provided by public health and assurance that the nurse will arrive in street clothes and an unmarked car may facilitate the referral.

The linkage of clients with service programs or agencies involves the mutual preparation of both client and resource. In addition, some follow-up may be required to ensure that the client actually made contact with the resource and that the initial contact lead to engagement in the program.

Preparing the service for the client may be as simple as providing pertinent information by telephone or on an appropriate referral form. (It is helpful and time saving to have a stock of frequently used forms on hand.) In cases where it is unclear whether or not the client is appropriate for the resource, a more complete assessment may be required. Some services have complex intake procedures and long waiting periods while others act quite quickly on more basic information.

As stated earlier, it is useful to describe the client in terms that fit the agency's criteria. It is also important not to be so creative in the presentation of the client that the agency feels manipulated to accept an inappropriate referral. Being honest about the difficulties which can be expected in serving the client enables the agency to be prepared to offer services appropriately and also enhances the ongoing relationship with the agency.

Preparing the client for the resource involves the same tasks. Pertinent information should be provided and the strengths and limitations of the service should be described honestly. For example, making a referral to "meals-on-wheels" and telling the client that someone will be bringing them a home-cooked meal and staying to chat while they eat will likely result in a dissatisfied client. Anyone who visits seniors in their homes can tell stories of homes where the meals delivered over several days are neatly stacked, untouched in the refrigerator or left to rot on the kitchen counter. The recipients may complain that the meat is too tough or the meal is unappealing. When asked why they do not cancel the service or try to request more satisfying meals, they often respond that their son or daughter or doctor wants them to continue. The link has been made—but not effectively.

The client's wishes should be clearly understood and acknowledged when describing a new service. It is usually more effective to anticipate some of the client's objections to a particular service and to talk about them in advance rather than to hope that the problems will not materialize. For example, a client expressed interest in attending a day program to give his wife some free time and to have some social life for himself. He had a disability which made him unable to participate in ordinary seniors' clubs so he was referred to a therapeutic day program. At the time of his referral, the day program had a large proportion of moderately demented clients. Rather than have the client arrive and quite accurately assess that he had nothing in common with the other participants, his worker discussed the situation before the first visit. Together, they were able to plan a strategy for him to meet his needs at the day centre despite the disabilities of the other clients.

TYPES OF RESOURCES

The following section outlines some of the types of services which are frequently useful in working with psychogeriatric clients.

Information Services

Community information centres are usually able to provide current information on services available within a specific community. They can often provide information about informal services as well as the specific services offered by established formal agencies. Information centres may publish guides which list a number of frequently called services. Libraries, public health departments, and hospital social work departments are other sources of information. These services are usually provided free of charge to the public with no restrictions on eligibility.

Assessments

In-home, out-patient, and in-patient assessments all have an important role in service delivery to seniors. In-home assessments are particularly important in determining the functional level of geriatric clients who may perform poorly in an unfamiliar setting or, conversely, may conceal their difficulties in maintaining their homes without assistance. In-patient assessment and treatment should be avoided unless clearly indicated. Older patients often lose functional abilities after a relatively short time away from their usual daily activities and routines, and may have difficulty resuming previous activities even after successful treatment. Out-patient assessments avoid the disruption of hospital admission and yet allow access to equipment and procedures which may not be available in the patient's home.

In most communities, home-based assessments can be arranged with public health nurses, visiting nurses (e.g. Victorian Order of Nurses), and family physicians. In addition, some communities have specialized geriatric and psychogeriatric programs which will provide assessment and consultation at home. Most assessment services are provided without cost to the individual. Visiting nurses charge a fee on a sliding scale. Eligibility criteria vary widely.

Continuing Treatment and Support

These services will usually be provided by the same agencies who perform the assessments stated earlier. Specialized psychogeriatric care may not be readily available in the community but consultation may be provided to visiting nurses, institutionally based staff, and others involved in long-term care. Again, these services are usually provided without cost to the individual or the fee may be adjusted to reflect the client's ability to pay.

Home-Help/Homemaking

These agencies provide a number of services to enable people with disabilities to continue to live in their own homes. Services range from cooking meals, light housework, and shopping to shovelling snow and home maintenance. The specific services offered by any particular agency are quite variable.

Home-help agencies tend to service a small defined neighborhood and may use volunteers to provide services. Home-help agencies usually charge a modest fee for their services and may offer a sliding scale. Homemaking agencies employ trained homemakers whose services may be covered by a government program such as Home Care. Fees may be adjusted according to income if the client is not eligible for fully funded services.

Day Hospitals/Day Programs

These programs may be designed for active treatment, rehabilitation, or long-term care. All provide opportunities for socialization. Day hospitals can be a very satisfactory way of providing necessary treatment and monitoring without the disruption of an in-patient admission. Alternatively, such partial hospitalization may allow an in-patient's stay to be shortened and provide for a gradual return to independent functioning.

Inadequate transportation services can be a serious barrier to the use of day programs. Many communities have some form of public transportation for the disabled but it is often inconvenient and unreliable. These services are usually described as curb-to-curb and, therefore, may be of no value to anyone who needs assistance getting out to the curb. Home-help agencies may provide transportation but have difficulty finding enough drivers to meet the needs. Thus, the need for and availability of appropriate transportation must be assessed. Day hospitals are usually free to the user but other day programs frequently charge a daily rate which may be prohibitive even in non-profit centres.

Recreation/Education Programs

Maintenance of good mental health generally requires that an individual be involved in interesting activities. Such activities may be solitary or social but should be stimulating to the individual. Municipal recreation departments, senior citizen centres, and educational institutions all provide programs which may be used by seniors. Often psychogeriatric clients need special assistance in fitting into regular programs. Many are not comfortable in group situations and need individualized programs which may be designed by an occupational therapist or a recreation specialist at a rehabilitation centre.

Financial/Legal Services

There is a myriad of financial programs available to seniors. However, seniors and their caregivers frequently do not take full advantage of the available support. Old Age Pension, Canada/Quebec Pensions, and company pensions are generally well known but must be applied for well in advance of the retirement date. The Guaranteed Income Supplement and its provincial counterparts are not always well understood. In addition, the Department of Veterans Affairs has a number of financial programs designed for veterans and their families. Municipal welfare departments will often assist with special needs even for people who are not receiving welfare. Financial support in the way of drug benefit cards, property tax rebates, subsidized housing, cost-free banking and reduced rates for almost everything can substantially reduce the cost of living for seniors who are sufficiently assertive to take advantage of their availability.

Older people have many of the same needs for legal services as do younger people and they have access to the same resources. In particular, older people are frequently concerned about power of attorney and wills. It is important that they get good legal advice to ensure that they have sufficient protection and to ensure that the people whom they trust with their affairs are indeed trustworthy. Most legal aid clinics will assist seniors in the preparation of simple wills and powers of attorney. It is the responsibility of a lawyer to ensure that the senior is competent to understand the issues being discussed and to make informed decisions.

For those who are unable to manage their own financial affairs, the Public Trustee, private trustees, family, and friends may be involved. The assessment of financial competence and these services are described further in Chapter 13. In summary, a geriatric client who is found incompetent to manage his or her finances may be quite vulnerable in the absence of appropriate guardianship. Incompetence may be temporary during an acute illness or permanent at some point in the course of dementia.

Support for Caregivers

This subject is addressed in more detail in Chapter 14, but needs to be mentioned here. Planning for support for the caregiver should be an integral part of any long-term care plan. Respite services which allow the caregiver a much needed break on a weekly basis as well as for holidays are essential. Often families organize respite amongst themselves but may need encouragement to do so. In many cases, there are no family or friends available and agency sponsored respite must be arranged. Respite care can usually be arranged in homes for the aged and retirement homes at its usual daily rate. Some chronic care hospitals provide respite care which is covered by the provincial health insurance plan. Community respite in the older person's home is rare but would be known to the information service in areas where it exists.

Family support groups can be invaluable for caregivers who are feeling alone with their concerns and frustrations. Family counselling agencies, mental health clinics or public health nurses may provide counselling for caregivers and seniors to enable them to cope more effectively with their problems. Specialized geriatric and psychogeriatric agencies frequently include support to family caregivers as part of their program.

Special Needs

There are a host of agencies and associations addressing the specific needs of people coping with particular problems and illnesses. The resources which they can provide should not be overlooked. The Alzheimer's Society, the Epilepsy Association, and the Stroke Recovery Association are a few of the many groups which may be able to provide information and services of use to the psychogeriatric client.

DEVELOPING RESOURCES

There is no community which offers all of the services that all of its residents might benefit from and certainly most commmunities fall far short of providing a full range of needed services. As one becomes more adept at finding and using existing community resources, one may also become very aware of and frustrated with the lack of particular services. One way to cope with this frustration is to become an advocate and an agent for change. Having identified one or more serious gaps in service, the worker then needs to identify others who may share this perception.

The development of a new service program is extremely difficult. Very often well-planned programs to meet clearly documented needs are not established simply because of lack of funds. Nevertheless, health care professionals should regard it as part of their mandate to contribute to service development. Some of the many steps involved in planning and implementing a new service are summarized below:

1. Identification of the need for a service.
2. Documentation of the location and potential number of clients who have the specific need.
3. Definition of the type of service required to meet the need.
4. Drafting a description of the proposed service. A written proposal usually requires the following elements: description of the need; description of the target population (demographic characteristics, potential numbers); description of the service objectives and how they will be met; staffing qualifications; and, budget (i.e. personnel, supplies, space).
5. Appeal to those who may assist in the implementation of the service (i.e. the general public, health care agencies, potential funding bodies).

Perhaps the greatest contribution that can be made by the individual health professional lies in the identification of patterns of unmet needs in a caseload.

CONCLUSION

Maintaining the psychogeriatric client in the community requires creative use of the full range of existing community resources. To do this requires detailed knowledge of the services available, a good understanding of clients' needs and preferences, and the time and inclination to ensure a good match between clients and services.

Providing a full opportunity for clients to achieve a good quality of life in the community often leads the health professional to the role of advocate. Encouraging agencies to expand their mandate to meet an identified need or working with others to develop a new service are important activities in ensuring that the needs of the psychiatrically impaired elderly are met.

REFERENCES AND SUGGESTED READINGS

Cole E. "Assessing Needs for Elders' Networks." *Journal of Gerontological Nursing*. 11: 731.

Connids I. March 1985. "The Service Needs of Older People: Implications for Public Policy." *Canadian Journal of Aging*. 4. 3.

Cox, F. M., J. L. Erlich, J. Rothman, and J. E. Tropman. (eds.) 1979. *Strategies of Community Organization*. 3rd ed. Itasca: F. E. Peacock Publishers, Inc.

Dunlop Burton D. May 1980. "Expanded Home-Based Care For the Impaired Elderly: Solution or Pipe Dream?" *American Journal of Public Health*. 70: 514.

Dunn R. B., L. MacBeath and D. Robertson. "Respite Admissions and The Disabled Elderly." *Journal of American Geriatrics Society*. 31: 613.

Lipsman Robbie et al. "Expanding Care for the Frail Aged at Home: An Imperative, An Opportunity." *New York University Education Quarterly*.

15

Community Psychiatry and Psychogeriatrics

Donald A. Wasylenki, M.D., M.Sc., F.R.C.P. (C)

Community psychiatry refers to the organized delivery of mental health services outside of traditional institutional settings. It also refers to the use of the community, that is, the community of professional and non-professional caregivers, in the treatment and prevention of mental illness. Practitioners emphasize social factors in the cause and course of mental illnesses, and the importance of the interpersonal environment in treatment. This approach attempts to understand symptoms as related to socially disruptive events or the absence of social support rather than to biochemical changes, intrapsychic conflicts, or faulty learning. Common biases include beliefs that it is better to be outside of a psychiatric hospital than in one; that good relationships are protective and sustaining; that activity is good; and that people who need support to live in the community should receive it. These fundamental aspects of community psychiatry are extremely important for the practice of psychogeriatrics.*

GENERAL PRINCIPLES

Community psychiatry received its greatest impetus from deinstitutional-ization. Two developments made deinstitutionalization possible. The first was the discovery of major tranquillizers which allowed psychotic patients to be treated outside of hospitals. Now concern has focussed on over-reliance on these drugs in community practice, and on their serious side effects, particularly

---

* This chapter has been adapted by permission from Chapter 8, "Community Psychiatry and Psychogeriatrics" in *Disturbed Behavior in the Elderly* by A. G. Awad, Henry B. Durost, H. M. Rosemary Meier and W. O. McCormick (eds.) Copyright 1986, Spectrum Publications, Inc., Jamaica, New York

in elderly patients. A study of psychiatric aftercare in Metropolitan Toronto revealed an alarming over-reliance on chemotherapy in the community management of discharged psychiatric patients, regardless of age. There was little evidence of comprehensive, rehabilitative programming. The second development was the recognition of the harmful effects of total institutional care. The syndrome of institutionalism is characterized by lack of initiative, apathy, withdrawal, submissiveness to authority, excessive dependence on the institution and feelings of worthlessness and dehumanization. Unfortunately the environments of many chronic care institutions, most of whose patients are elderly and physically disabled, seem tailor-made to induce this syndrome. Its manifestations are readily and immediately apparent in the lounges, hallways and rooms of many nursing homes, homes for the aged, and chronic care hospitals. Important components of sociotherapy such as patient self-government, large and small group meetings and other stimulants to socialization are rarely systematically practised in geriatric institutions. These institutions suffer from a lack of mental health expertise, even though extremely high percentages of residents are mentally ill.

The social deterioration found in hospitalized psychiatric patients has been described as the social breakdown syndrome. This refers to the lack of interpersonal skills and other competencies through induction into a devalued role with low expectations of normal human behavior. Others have argued that the social breakdown syndrome provides a model for understanding normal ageing in most western societies. The elderly person, by virtue of being old, is labelled as useless and deviant, like the chronically mentally ill patient. There are few roles, behavioral norms or reference groups for the elderly, and those that do exist are pegged to middle age. Thus, an increased sensitivity to external cues for behavior develops. Since most of these cues are negative, that is, elderly people are not really expected to do anything, feelings of uselessness and low self-worth develop, and complementary behaviors evolve. This results in loss of skills and competencies in a way analogous to what is observed in institutionalized patients. Here, however, not only are the elderly people in nursing homes or other institutional settings being described, but also the elderly people living in the community. Analysis of the pathogenesis of the social breakdown syndrome leads to broad social strategies for intervention to produce a cycle of social re-integration. This must be based upon challenging beliefs that self-worth is tied to productivity, the development of effective roles for elderly citizens, especially in consultative areas, and the expectation that elderly people will continue to direct their own lives. These strategies arise from normalizing psychosocial approaches to the thousands of chronic psychiatric patients discharged into unprepared communities.

Community psychiatry continues to learn important lessons from its failures. Data indicate that one year after hospital discharge, 40 to 50 percent of patients have been re-admitted. Within three to five years recidivism increases to 75 percent. Only 10 to 30 percent of patients ever become competitively employed after discharge. These poor outcomes are rooted in the diagnostic system and intervention techniques utilized in the delivery of mental health services to the chronically mentally ill. Traditional psychiatric diagnoses and traditional in-patient and out-patient treatment techniques have little impact on outcomes for disabled patients. What has developed is a rehabilitation model to complement the traditional treatment model. Treatment is for signs and symptoms; rehabilitation is for disability. Many chronic mental patients and many psychogeriatric patients are disabled as a result of mental illness. More than diagnosis and treatment, they require skills and support to function in the community environments of their choice. This requires an approach grounded in the fields of physical rehabilitation and psychotherapy. This approach must emphasize patient skills and deficits, it must be environment specific and it must involve the patient in the entire process. It means, as stated by Anthony, that practitioners must ensure that

> the person with a psychiatric disability possesses those physical, emotional and intellectual skills necessary to live, learn and work in his particular environment. The major rehabilitative interventions involve either helping patients to acquire or apply particular skills they need to function in their environment and/or developing environmental resources needed to support or strengthen the patient's assessed level of functioning (1978, 368).

There is evidence now that rehabilitative techniques can improve outcomes in chronically disabled patients. This is an extremely important lesson to be learned from community psychiatry. Diagnosis and treatment is not enough. Rehabilitation must follow.

Lamb (1982) has outlined other obstacles to successful deinstitutionalization, many of which are applicable to the problems of psychogeriatric patients. First, there has been a failure to recognize that there are many different kinds of long-term patients who vary greatly in their capacity for improvement. Secondly, there has been a failure to understand that long-term patients also vary in their motivation to change. Thirdly, professionals have been slow to understand that in the absence of adequate social support networks, treatment gains in psychosocial functioning are seldom maintained after completion of programs. Finally, treatment goals have too often been biased in terms of acceptable functioning for white, professional, middle-class, middle aged patients. Lamb (1982) concludes that real progress will be made in the treatment of long-term disability only when it is realized that simply improving the quality of life and providing comfortable living in a non-hospital environment are acceptable therapeutic goals. In working with the severely disabled elderly, these are indeed significant objectives.

One proposed solution to the problem of the chronic patient in the community has been to identify model programs whenever they develop and then to mass produce these programs everywhere. There are, of course, various and obvious reasons why this approach is unlikely to be successful. However, Bachrach (1980) has conceptualized eight elementary principles common to successful model programs which should be of interest to psychogeriatric service providers. They are as follows: (1) Assign top priority to the care of the most severely impaired. In psychogeriatrics this means assigning top priority to patients and families struggling with progressive dementing illness. (2) Establish realistic linkages with other resources in the community. Given the multi-dimensional nature of much of psychogeriatric disability, this principle is extremely important. (3) Provide out-of-hospital alternatives for the full range of functions performed in hospital settings. With the psychogeriatric population, this often involves a more intensive supervisory function provided by family and/or neighbors in consultation with psychogeriatric specialists and case managers. (4) Individually tailor treatment for each patient. This must always be based upon a comprehensive psychogeriatric assessment carried out by a psychogeriatric specialist. (5) Determine cultural relevance and specificity. This means tailoring programs to conform to the local realities of the community in which they are located. This implies knowledge of ethno-cultural aspects of ageing and of the resources available in any given program area. (6) Employ trained staff who are attuned to the unique survival problems of the elderly psychiatrically impaired patient. Program staff must be carefully trained in techniques specific to psychogeriatric case management, for example the management of urinary incontinence and amnesia. (7) Provide access to a complement of hospital beds. In the psychogeriatric area, relief beds are often more appropriate so as to support the exhausted family caretaker for short periods. (8) Establish an ongoing internal assessment mechanism that permits continuous self-monitoring.

SERVICE COMPONENTS

What is the rationale for providing community-based care for the mentally ill elderly?

First of all, given the expanding elderly population and the high prevalence of psychiatric disorder, there can never be enough institutional beds to treat everyone. In addition, elderly people prefer treatment at home, and they tend to avoid contact with institutional services. It is widely recognized that elderly people should be moved from their homes only after careful consideration of alternatives. Relocation of elderly patients often has deleterious effects, including anxiety, depression, confusion, and even death. And it has been shown that in areas that provide adequate community support, a significantly higher proportion of ill people can be accommodated at home.

Given that there is an adequate rationale for community treatment, what are the important components?

An adequate community-based service delivery system must provide both specialist and case management functions. Core specialist functions include assessment and planning, consultation, and education. Core case management functions include planning, linking, monitoring, and advocating.

Specialist Functions

Assessment

One of the most important skills of a psychogeriatric specialist is the ability to carry out a comprehensive diagnostic and functional assessment and to develop a management plan. Community-based treatment programs must provide high quality assessments in home and other community settings if they are to reach the patient population and to achieve acceptability. A very important part of the selection and training of professionals seeking to become psychogeriatric specialists should involve assessment skills. It has been suggested that

> competencies needed to accomplish the psychogeriatric assessment in a home setting include the ability to inspire trust, gain entry, perform a skilful interview and a screening physical exam, document a mental status, assess the environmental and supportive network and the coping abilities of the individual in relation to activities of daily living, and determine the individual's economic situation (Dagon 1982, 139).

It is also extremely important to be able to arrange for immediate hands on care or treatment.

It should be emphasized that this is a clinical assessment which should always be carried out by a clinician who specializes in the assessment of psychogeriatric problems. These assessment skills are not exclusively physician competencies. For example, experienced psychiatric nurse-clinicians are able to function very effectively as psychogeriatric specialists. Almost all psychogeriatric diagnoses should be based on clinical criteria. Laboratory tests and specialized procedures such as computerized tomography must be available for a small percentage of cases, but day-to-day familiarity with these techniques is not essential to the assessment function. The clinical examination of the patient is by far the most important feature, and professionals trained in psychogeriatric clinical assessment are the only people who should perform this extremely important function. The ongoing treatment plan and the case management functions rest upon assessment findings.

Training for assessment includes the phenomenology and presentation of the major mental disorders that occur in the elderly. There must be a clear understanding of the three-fold purpose of any assessment, that is, to obtain data, to establish rapport, and to involve the patient. The psychogeriatric specialist must understand normal ageing, in particular, phenomena such as benign or senescent forgetfulness, slowing of reaction time, and decreased stress responsiveness. The recognition of anticipatory, normal and pathological grief, and the particular forms grief takes among the elderly is essential. The specialist must be aware that depression is extremely common in the elderly and in a high percentage of cases goes untreated. S/he must be able to recognize typical affective disorders, depressive pseudodementia, masked depressions, and delusional depressions. In other words, s/he must be familiar with the protean presentations of affective disorders in late life, and also with the life events which commonly precipitate them. In dealing with dementia, s/he must be able to assess the major features of cognitive impairment including diminished memory, disorientation, shallow affect, impaired judgment, and intellectual deterioration, as well as to recognize more subtle early signs. S/he must be aware of catastrophic reactions in demented patients to relocation to institutional settings. S/he must be able to distinguish acute confusional states from dementia and be aware of the common causes of delirium in the elderly. S/he must recognize and differentiate various paranoid presentations such as paranoid forgetfulness, paranoid delirium and late paraphrenia, and s/he must be familiar with characteristic reactions to chronic and catastrophic physical illnesses. S/he must have a working knowledge of the effects and side effects of common medications prescribed for elderly patients. In particular, s/he must recognize neuroleptic-induced syndromes, inadequate doses of antidepressant medication and harmful dependencies on alcohol and/or minor tranquillizers. This is to give some idea of the expertise necessary.

The other aspect of the assessment is the functional or rehabilitative component. A psychogeriatric assessment is not complete simply because a diagnosis has been made. It is necessary to describe in detail which important activities the patient can or cannot do. This part of the assessment should be based on skill strengths and deficits and should be environment specific. For example, in considering whether a mildly demented elderly person can remain at home, it is necessary to know whether s/he can safely operate the stove or whether s/he is able to regularly find her/his way to a grocery store. If s/he has deficits in these areas, then her/his environment could be augmented through a "meals-on-wheels" intervention. All important activities of daily living, basic and instrumental, should be assessed from a strengths-deficits perspective. It is often surprising to discover a significant degree of positive cognition in patients diagnosed as suffering from dementia.

There are a number of instruments available to assist with the psychogeriatric assessment, and specialists should be familiar with these. The two most common multi-dimensional instruments are the OARS (Older American Resources and Services) and the CARE (Comprehensive Assessment and Referral Evaluation). Both of these cover social, economic, mental and physical functioning, and activities of daily living. The CARE emphasizes mental health issues, particularly screening scales for dementia and depression. For assessing depression in the elderly the Zung Scale or the Beck Depression Inventory may be useful. The Mental Status Questionnaire or the Mini Mental State Examination provide a quick measure of the state of the demented patient and the Global Deterioration Scale has been recommended for more precise staging. Finally, for the assessment of functional psychoses, the Brief Psychiatric Rating Scale is useful. There are a number of Activities of Daily Living Scales available and Anthony (1980) has published a useful workbook on rehabilitation diagnosis.

Consultation

The second important specialist function is psychogeriatric consultation. Mental health consultation is one of the cornerstones of community psychiatric practice. Given the high prevalence of severe mental disorder in the community as a result of deinstitutionalization, and the scarcity of trained professionals to deal directly with all severely disordered patients, consultation has developed as a means to achieve a multiplier effect. A consultant, who is a specialist, is able to assist numbers of consultees and through them their clients by using a specific form of interaction. Mental health consultation does not simply mean that psychiatrists tell other people what to do. The term "consultation" should be used in a restricted sense to denote the process of interaction between two professional persons; the consultant who is a specialist, and the consultee, who invokes help in regard to a current work problem with which the latter is having some difficulty, and which s/he has decided is within the former's area of specialized competence. The work problem involves the management or treatment of one or more clients of the consultee, or the planning or implementation of a program to cater to such clients.

There are several reasons why it is important for psychogeriatric specialists to learn techniques of mental health consultation. First is the very high prevalence of severe mental disorder in the elderly, estimated in the range of 15 to 20 percent. Second is the scarcity of well-trained psychogeriatric personnel. Training programs for psychiatric residents have only just begun to develop in North America. Psychiatrists, in general practice, devote very little time to elderly patients. Despite the fact that the elderly constitute nearly one-tenth of the population and have a higher incidence and prevalence of mental disorder than other age groups, fewer than 4 percent of psychiatric out-patients are 65 or older. Psychiatrists in private practice give an estimated two percent of their time to the elderly. In Ontario in 1979, only 4.75 percent of Ontario Hospital Insurance Plan billings for out-patient psychiatric services were for people over age 65. It is also true that elderly patients under-utilize mental health services that are available to them. They may associate psychiatric assistance only with very severe mental impairment, or they may feel unwelcome at out-patient clinics. They may also fear that the more service contacts they have, the more likely they are to end up in an institution. However, as the Group for the Advancement of Psychiatry's report on the Aged and Community Mental Health emphasized, the normal dependencies of the elderly lead large numbers of them to seek help from many different agencies, and these agencies and their personnel should be the locus of mental health consultation. These include home care programs, senior citizen centres, family physicians, nursing homes, and homes for the aged. In Metropolitan Toronto, for example, most home health care services are provided through the Home Care Program for Metropolitan Toronto. Services include nursing, physiotherapy, occupational therapy, speech therapy, and visiting homemaking. Since 1975 when Home Care was made available to patients in nursing homes and homes for the aged, roughly 60 percent of all home care services were delivered to patients over age 65. In 1980 (Annual Report of the Homecare Program per Metropolitan Toronto), 12 597 elderly patients were seen, and 20 percent of patients in the program were 80 years and older. In addition, in Metropolitan Toronto there are roughly 12 000 elderly residents in nursing homes, homes for the aged, and chronic care hospitals. It is these programs, institutions, and personnel who should be the recipients of expert psychogeriatric consultation.

An essential aspect of consultation is that the professional responsibility for the client remains with the consultee who is free to accept or reject the consultant's help. Action emerging from the consultation is the responsibility of the consultee. Another essential aspect is that the consultant acts not only to help with a particular case, but also to add to the knowledge and skills of the consultee. So the technique provides an opportunity for a small number of consultants to exert a widespread effect in any system of care.

There are four fundamental types of mental health consultation, all of which are essential for the psychogeriatric specialist. These four types have become known as client-centred case consultation, consultee-centred case consultation, program-centred administrative consultation, and consultee-centred administrative consultation. Each type is associated with characteristic technical demands upon the consultant. There is a need to provide consultation to residential facilities run by administrators and staff not specifically trained in the management of psychiatric patients. Principles apply to work in nursing homes, homes for the aged, chronic care hospitals, and senior citizens' residences. The consultant must be familiar with the facilities' operating procedures, with the various and diverse needs of individual patients and with the administration's attitude toward mental health professionals. The consultant must be aware of problems that arise when s/he provides both consultative and direct services in the same facility. Consultants may advise administrators on issues such as determining admission criteria, understanding the mental health system and handling a variety of difficult behaviors. Nursing homes present particular problems for psychogeriatric consultants. Psychiatric disturbances are probably the predominant form of illness in nursing homes, and yet psychiatric expertise is seldom available. One goal must be to demonstrate that specific therapies for specific disorders found among nursing home patients are both effective and economically feasible. In addition, efforts must be directed at upgrading the psychogeriatric knowledge and skill of nursing home staff.

Education

The third core specialist function is education. Education is differentiated from consultation in that the specialist has a set body of knowledge to impart, and students are not free to accept or reject content. Many community practitioners working with elderly patients are limited by deficiencies in basic clinical knowledge. Knowledge however, is a prerequisite for effective utilization of consultation. Thus it is necessary for psychogeriatric specialists to develop effective educational programs. These should include courses covering topics in clinical geriatric psychiatry, such as: normal ageing, depression in the elderly, late life dementias, acute confusional states, reactions to chronic illness, paranoid states, medications and the elderly, assessment, management principles, and family supports. They should also include courses in techniques such as grief counselling and community service co-ordination. The content of this handbook has been designed to address these specific issues.

Case Management Functions

The second important service component is psychogeriatric case management. The case manager is the person who is involved with the patient in an ongoing personal and therapeutic relationship as the management plan is implemented over time. In most cases the case management function should not be carried out by the psychogeriatric specialist.

The concept of case management was developed as a way to help chronically mentally ill patients adjust to the community by providing a continuity of care agent. It was felt that because these patients are faced with fragmented, unco-ordinated, competitive and often unresponsive services to meet their needs, what was required was a new kind of mental health worker, called a case manager, who would help the individual patient navigate the often confusing community service network. The functions of case management vary with different programs and different authors but usually include the following: planning activities and services with and for the patient; linking or connecting patients to appropriate programs, agencies or services; monitoring patient progress during treatment; advocating with the various components of the management package on the patient's behalf; and reviewing and updating the initial patient management plan with the patient and/or other professionals. In some models, the assessment function is added to case management, but experience suggests that it is more advantageous to separate these functions, at least until one has identified case managers who are clearly able to function at the assessment level.

A psychogeriatric case manager should participate, with a psychogeriatric specialist, in the initial assessment and development of the management plan. This is often a consultative relationship. Ongoing help to the patient is provided in making concrete plans, finding and gaining access to appropriate programs or services, checking regularly with the patient and the program with regard to progress, helping to sort out problems the patient might be encountering with program components such as family doctors, visiting homemakers, or "meals-on-wheels", and reviewing plans with the patient and the specialist.

Psychogeriatric case managers may be public health nurses who carry out a number of other functions as well, but who have a special interest in the elderly. They may be home visiting occupational therapists, family physicians, relatives, neighbors, or volunteers. These particular functions may be better carried out by non-credentialled professionals selected on the basis of personality traits, interests, and motivation rather than on background education and experience. It is the ability to work closely with the psychogeriatric specialist and to establish a friendly, co-operative relationship with the elderly patient that is most important. It is not necessary for the case manager to establish a traditional therapeutic relationship with the patient. On the other hand, more than just a broker of services is necessary. The nature of the relationship will vary with specific program objectives and case managers themselves.

The Psychiatrist

What is the role of the psychiatrist who has specialized in psychogeriatrics within a community-based service delivery system? It is not the psychiatrist's role to do routine community assessments and/or case management. Because s/he is a very rare commodity, s/he should be available to assist with difficult cases and to provide ongoing training for a staff of psychogeriatric specialists and case managers. Involvement in administrative and evaluative research within an integrated service program is also desirable. S/he should provide an ongoing review of the work of the psychogeriatric specialists. Another important function is to help non-physician colleagues feel comfortable in dealing with the many other physicians and psychiatrists involved in the care of elderly patients. Above all, the psychiatrist should be an educator and an advocate on behalf of the elderly who are mentally ill.

SOCIAL NETWORKS

Social isolation or impaired social relations are common features of the chronically mentally ill and of psychogeriatric patients. For both groups, much of the planning by specialists and much of the case management involves strengthening social supports.

One's relationships have the potential to provide both enduring and short-term support. This support consists of both emotional support and task-oriented assistance provided by an individual's social network. According to Caplan (1974), systems may operate in two ways: (1) They collect and store information and provide guidance and direction for an individual in a stressful situation. (2) They act as a refuge or sanctuary to which an individual may return for rest and recuperation in-between sorties into a stressful environment.

Caplan (1974) has provided a classification of natural support systems. The basic support system consists of "kith and kin"—a person's close friends and relatives. Ideally they provide ongoing guidance and direction and also sustain their members in acute crisis situations. Often however, because of the specific demands of a particular crisis, kith and kin supports may be augmented by the special services of people in the community described as informal caregivers. Informal caregivers may be "generalists" or "specialists". Generalists are people who are widely recognized as having wisdom in matters of human relationships. They are people whose advice has been good in the past and so have earned and maintained a local reputation as helpful. Specialists are people who have successfully coped with some hazardous life event and are sought out by others who find themselves in the same situation. The outstanding characteristics of these informal caregivers are that they are non-professionals and that there is a mutual and reciprocal quality in their interactions with the people they help. Helping others often reinforces and restores their own feelings of mastery.

The organizational counterparts of individual caregivers are voluntary service groups and specific self-help organizations. Caplan (1974) also argues that religious dominations are usually the most widely available organized support systems in any community. They are organized into congregations of neighbors. They hold regular meetings. There is a shared theology and a common value system. Members are enjoined to help each other. Service programs are provided at predictable crisis times such as birth, marriage, illness, and death.

Turning to specific components of social support the confidant is of crucial importance. A confidant is defined as a person with whom an individual has a close, intimate and confiding relationship. Such a relationship must be characterized by availability, self-disclosure, and reciprocity. Intimacy is an important variable influencing adjustment to hazardous life events in old age.

Community psychiatry has focussed on the notion of social networks as a way of operationalizing the concept of social support. One's social network simply refers to the number and arrangement of potentially supportive people in one's life.

Neurotics have been shown to have smaller networks than normals. The neurotic's pattern of relationships resembles a wheel with no connections between the spokes. Neurotics also have more negative relationships than normals. Psychotic patients have severely impoverished networks consisting of four to five members who are usually family. Their networks tend to be very dense and are described as binding. Studies have confirmed that network size tends to decrease with increasing severity and chronicity of psychiatric conditions. In addition, correlations have been found between network size and structure and length of community-tenure and rehospitalization rates.

As a result of these and other findings, analysis of chronic patients' social networks is becoming an important aspect of community practice. Several mapping approaches are currently available to assist with planning interventions. Such interventions include social network therapy, devised social networks and co-ordinated social networks.

Social network therapy refers to the assembly of the natural social network including family members and significant others, to affect beneficial change for the patient. This usually results in a network nucleus emerging consisting of people who are willing to actively participate as problem-solvers, support agents, and communication links to help the patient during a crisis. Social network therapy thus tries to actualize the supportive potential in the patient's natural social network.

Devised social networks are organized to perform specific functions for patients lacking natural social networks. Such functions may include shopping, cooking, or cleaning. These functions may be performed by mental health professionals, community agencies, religious congregations, self-help groups, neighborhood figures, students, or volunteers. Devising social networks for isolated patients is a crucial case management skill if community adjustment is to be maintained. At times, the members of such networks, who often will not know one another, need to be assembled by the case manager in the same way as the natural social network.

Regardless of the type of social network involved in a particular case, a mental health worker needs to co-ordinate the network at the community level. In some cases, co-ordination involves only the natural social network; in others it involves only the devised social network. Ideally however, both types of network, working together, is the optimal solution. It is usually the responsibility of the case manager to mobilize and co-ordinate these networks. Linking patients with sources of support, either natural or devised, and then linking the links is the essence of the social network approach.

With regard to social networks and the elderly, being married or employed, or having substantial social activity (participation) protects against low morale in old age. In a sample of 280 people aged 63 and older, 83 percent of those with low social interaction were depressed whereas only 42 percent of those with high social interaction were depressed. More recently in a national probability survey of the non-institutionalized elderly, the immediate family of the old person was shown to be the major social support in time of illness and the extended family was the main tie for the elderly to the community. The main source of help for bedridden people is the husband or wife. The main community ties for the elderly who are well are regular, concerned visits from members of the kin network. This is in keeping with the concept of intermittent and continuous support. Also elderly people who require activities of daily living support to live independently rely on informal support networks such as relatives, friends, and neighbors rather than formal ones such as community agencies. Spouses are the primary source of help for the married elderly and daughters are the major helpers when the spouse is not present or when the level of support provided by the spouse is not sufficient. Informal helping networks increase in both size and scope as functional capacities decline.

A review of 153 elderly first admissions to a psychiatric hospital found that few needed to be hospitalized had the available social supports (especially the family and kin network) been utilized. The loss of interpersonal support is highly significant in the development of mental illness in the elderly, particularly depression. Social support systems may determine whether or not an elderly person becomes institutionalized. These supports include family, friends, work and job associations, interest groups and other local caregivers who provide self-esteem, intimacy, and solidarity.

The size of the North American family is decreasing so that there are fewer young people to support the elderly. The older relative in question is more apt to be a woman, a widow, and very old. Three-quarters of men over 65 live with spouses whereas only one-third of women do. Daughters usually take care of elderly widows but fewer daughters are available now as many are in the labor force. There is a tremendous need for support services to assist families and other natural network members to carry on with relatives at home. Network breakdown most commonly occurs when the person providing most of the home support can no longer cope, often due to the development of disturbed sleep or incontinence in the elderly relative.

Important factors leading to institutionalization are not having a family member, having a family member who is unavailable, or a child who is alienated. Comparing like groups in and out of institutions, the most significant difference is the availability of social support in the form of a family. It is also important to realize that when it does become necessary to institutionalize an elderly relative, the family will require assistance from either the case manager or the psychogeriatric specialist. The decision to institutionalize a parent has been called the nadir in the life of any individual. It precipitates serious conflicts in the patient's natural social network which have the potential to impair family decision-making and to create lasting animosity and family disruption. It is important to help families identify what is essentially a grief reaction in the pre-institutional period.

Contacts at work may be second in importance only to family contacts in a person's social network. Work can be an important source of non-familial social and interpersonal activities. An important network intervention may involve linking a recent retiree with volunteer services to enable him to regain lost interaction while engaging in beneficial work. Red Cross, hospital services, friendly visitors, and meals-on-wheels are examples.

There is a pressing need for community services. These are the components of devised social networks. The most useful services in preventing institution-alization of the elderly are home-care services and visiting homemakers. All that may be required is a few hours help, two to three days per week to maintain an elderly couple comfortably at home. Similarly, meal services can make a very significant difference. For relatives supporting demented patients at home, respite services are very cost-effective. Many families can cope for extended periods of time if they can look forward to some rest by having an institution provide care for a short period. Once again, the important function of any community-based psychogeriatric service is co-ordination of both natural and devised social networks. This enables elderly people who require support to obtain it. This is not to say however that there are no limitations. For the elderly person who is severely demented and who has no significant family support, maintenance in the community through a devised social network may be neither humane nor possible. In addition, family support of the elderly, although beneficial for the old person, may impose a heavy burden on the family. Difficulties arise from the physical and mental condition of the patient and fatigue, anxiety and lack of information among family caregivers. On the other hand, the vast majority of family caregivers report many satisfying aspects of caring for dependent elderly relatives at home. The greater fault among psychogeriatric service providers usually lies on the side of inadequate recognition of the supportive potential available to many elderly patients, and in the inability to support available caregivers and to recruit new personnel in order to devise new programs where they are needed.

REFERENCES AND SUGGESTED READINGS

Anthony W. A., M. R. Cohen and R. Vitalo. 1978. "The Measurement of Rehabilitation Out-come." *Schizophrenia Bulletin.* 4: 365.

Anthony W. A. and R. R. Carkhuff. 1978. "The Functional Professional Therapeutic Agent." *Effective Psychotherapy: A Handbook of Research.* Ed. A. S. Gurman and A. M. Razin. Oxford: Pergamon Press.

Anthony W. A. 1980. *The Principles of Psychiatric Rehabilitation.* Baltimore: University Park Press.

Bachrach L. L. 1980. "Overview: Model Programs for Chronic Mental Patients." *American Journal of Psychiatry.* 137: 1023.

Blau Z. S. 1973. *Old Age in a Changing Society: New Viewpoints.* New York.

Brothwood J. 1971. "The Organization and Development of Services for the Aged with Special Reference to the Mentally Ill." *Recent Developments in Psychogeriatrics.* British Journal of Psychiatry Special Publication No. 6.

Brown G. W. and T. Harris. 1978. *Social Origins of Depression.* London: Tavistock.

Butler R. N. 1975. "Psychiatry and the Elderly: An Overview." *American Journal of Psychiatry.* 132: 893.

Caplan G. 1970. *The Theory and Practice of Mental Health Consultation.* New York: Basic Books.

Caplan G. 1963. "Types of Mental Health Consultation." *American Journal of Orthopsychiatry.* 33: 470.

Caplan G. 1974. *Support Systems and Community Mental Health.* New York: Behavioural Publications.

Cohen G. D. 1976. "Mental Health Services and the Elderly: Needs and Options." *American Journal of Psychiatry.* 133: 65.

Dagon E. M. 1982. "Planning and Development Issues in Implementing Community-Based Mental Health Services for the Elderly." *Hospital and Community Psychiatry.* 33: 137.

Garetz F. K. 1975. "The Psychiatrist's Involvement With Aged Patients." *American Journal of Psychiatry.* 132: 63.

Group for the Advancement of Psychiatry, Committee on Aging. 1971. *The Aged and Community Mental Health: A Guide to Program Development.* Vol. VIII. Report No. 81.

Gruenberg E. M., D. M. Turns and S. P. Segal et al. 1972. "Social-Breakdown Syndrome: Environmental and Host Factors Associated with Chronicity." *American Journal of Public Health.* 62: 91.

Kasl S. F. 1972. "Physical and Mental Health Effects of Involuntary Relocation and Institutionalization of the Elderly—A Review." *American Journal of Public Health.* 62: 377.

Kuypers J. and V. Bengston. 1973. "Social Breakdown and Competence." *Human Development.* 16: 181.

Lamb H. R. 1982. *Treating the Long-Term Mentally Ill.* San Francisco: Jossey-Bass.

Lamb H. R. and C. L. Peterson. 1983. "The New Community Consultation." *Hospital and Community Psychiatry.* 34: 59.

Lowenthal M. F. and C. Haven. 1968. "Interaction and Adaptation: Intimacy As A Critical Variable." *American Sociological Review.* 33: 20.

Myers J. M. and C. S. Drayer. 1979. "Support Systems and Mental Illness in the Elderly." *Community Mental Health Journal.* 15: 277.

Ontario Ministry of Health. 1978. *Report of the Ontario Council of Health, Health Care for the Aged.*

Pattison E. M., R. Llamas and G. Hurd. 1979. "Social Network Mediation of Anxiety." *Psychiatric Annals.* 9: 56.

Roth M. and C. O. Mountjoy. 1980. "Mental Health Services for the Elderly Living in the Community: A United Kingdom Perspective." *International Journal of Mental Health.* 8: 6.

Sainsbury P. and J. Grad De Alarcon. 1973. "Evaluating A Service in Sussex." *Roots of Evaluation: The Epidemiological Basis for Planning Psychiatric Services.* Ed. J. K. Wing and H. Hafner. London: Oxford University Press.

Shanas E. 1979. "The Family As A Social Support System in Old Age." *The Gerontologist.* 19: 169.

Stotsky B. A. 1967. "Psychiatric Disorders Common to Psychiatric and Non-psychiatric Patients in Nursing Homes." *Journal of American Geriatrics Society.* 15: 644.

Turkat D. 1980. "Social Networks: Theory and Practice." *Journal of Community Psychology.* 8: 99.

Wasylenki D., P. Goering and W. Lancee et al. 1981. "Psychiatric Aftercare: Identified Needs Versus Referral Patterns." *American Journal of Psychiatry.* 138: 1228.

Weissman M. W. and J. K. Myers. 1979. "Depression in the Elderly: Research Directions in Psychopathology, Epidemiology and Treatment." *Journal of Geriatric Psychiatry.* 12: 187.

Wing J. K. and B. Morris. 1981. "Clinical Basis of Rehabilitation." *Handbook of Psychiatric Rehabilitation Practice.* Ed. J. K. Wing and B. Morris. Oxford: Oxford University Press.

Index

List of figures

List of tables

The Science and Practice of Gerontology:

A Multidisciplinary Approach

Nancy J. Osgood and Ann H.L. Sontz

1989 ISBN 1 85302 044 3

The Science and Practice of Gerontology provides a definitive reference guide for issues of theory, research, and practice in gerontology. The articles deal with the psychological, social, and cultural domains affecting older people, and also covers general biomedical understandings and practical/clinical applications. The contributors broadly outline the most relevant academic issues, including cross-cultural perspectives on age and ageing; past and future trends in life expectancy with underlying explanations; innovations and advances in research design and methodology i the study of the ageing process and the effects of age as a variable; and past and current theoretical perspectives on the psychology and sociology of ageing. Concerns pertinent for practitioners and clinicians are addressed, such as successful counselling therapies with older adults and changes in social work and rehabilitation practice with the elderly. A wide-sweeping multidisciplinary review of a rapidly expanding field of interest is provided, reflecting a definite desire among the contributors to evolve a theoretical apparatus and a related, applied arena of endeavour. An extraordinarily detailed reference, this work will be a valuable resource for gerontologists, social workers, psychologists, and doctors specialising in geriatrics.

CONTENTS Foreword, T. Franklin Williams. Preface. Acknowledgements. 1. Introduction. Within and Beyond the Academy: Backgrounds to Gerontology Research and Practice, Ann H L Sontz. PART I. SCIENCE IN GERONTOLOGY. 2. The Biology of Ageing, Edward J Masoro. 3. The Psychology of Adult Development and Ageing: New Approaches and Methodologies in the Developmental Study of Cognition and Personality, William J Hoyer and Karen Hooker. 4. Theory and Research in Social Gerontology, Nancy J Osgood. 5. Whither Anthropological Gerontology? Barbara Hornum and Anthony P Glascock. PART II. THE PRACTICING DISCIPLINES. 6. The Relationship of Geriatrics and Gerontology: On Forging Links Between Curing and Caring, Evan Calkins and Jurgis Karuza. 7. Background to Counselling the Elderly: Perspectives from Counselling Psychology, Roselle Acerno Kalosieh and Joseph Pedoto. 8. Social Work and Ageing, Louis Lowy. 9. Afterword. Facing the Frontiers: Interdisciplinary Issues and Agendas, Joan B Wood, Iris A Parham, and Jodi L Teitelman. Index.

Victims of Confusion:

Case Studies of Elderly Sufferers from Confusion and Dementia

Alyson Leslie

1990 128 pages ISBN 1 85302 040 0

Case Studies for Practice 5

This book describes the experiences of a number of elderly sufferers and their carers. The experience of people in residential respite care is also discussed as well as experiences in local authority and hospital day care settings.

Contents: 1. Confusion and Dementia - the Quiet Crisis. 2. Types of Provision and Characteristics of Users. 3. Caring for the Carers. 4. Case Studies of Sufferers Living Alone. 5. Case Studies of Sufferers Living with Carers. 6. Reactions to Respite and Day Care. 7. Managing Crises. 8. Support Networks. 9. Models of Intervention. 10. Outcomes and Indicators.

Structuring the Therapeutic Process: Compromise with Chaos
The Therapist's Response to the Individual and the Group
Murray Cox
1988 ISBN 1 85302 028 1
'...outstanding...derived from unusually diverse experience...a literate, wise and witty book. It is also eclectic. Dr Cox has gathered a rich harvest from many sources.'
- American Journal of Psychiatry

Coding the Therapeutic Process: Emblems of Encounter
A Manual for Counsellors and Therapists
Murray Cox
1988 ISBN 1 85302 029 X
A manual of visual display systems which suggests various forms of notation for recording a patient's kinship network, his living conditions and life events alongside his clinical history. It also indicates ways of recording inner and outer world phenomenon.

Dramatherapy with Families and Groups: A Handbook for Social Workers and Therapists
Sue Jennings
1990 ISBN 1 85302 014 1
The book provides a working framework for dramatherapists, social workers, family and marital therapists, and others running groups. This framework primarily deals with dramatherapy in the non-clinical setting such as family centres, residential children's homes, social services resources and intermediate treatment centres.

Art Therapy and Dramatherapy: Their Relation and Practice
Sue Jennings and Ase Minde
1990 ISBN 1 85302 027 3

Drama and Healing:
The Roots of Drama Therapy
Roger Grainger
1990 ISBN 1 85302 048 6
The author uses a particular psychological approach to understanding the therapeutic process involved in drama - namely, personal construct psychology. He argues that personal construct theory provides a hermeneutically useful approach to the study of drama therapy. He shows that drama therapy itself is an effective treatment for depression and schizophrenia, having a measurable effect on thought disorder.

Storymaking in Education and Therapy
Alida Gersie and Nancy King
1990

Storymaking in Bereavement
Alida Gersie
1990

Art Therapy in Practice
Edited by Marian Liebmann
1990 ISBN 1 85302 057 5
ISBN 1 85302 058 3 paper
Introduction. 1. Images of Self, John Ford. 2. Art Psychotherapy, the Search for Meaning, and Manic Depression, Roy Thornton. 3. The Revolving Door (Art Therapy in groups with people who have had long experience of the psychiatric services), Claire Skailes. 4. A Place to Be - art therapy and community-based rehabilitation, Sarah Lewis. 5. Swimming Upstream - Art Therapy with the Psycho-geriatric Population in One Health District, Karen Drucker. 6. An Integrative Approach to Art Therapy with Children, Tish Feilden. 7. Art Therapy - a Medium of Self-Discovery and Development for People with Mental Handicap, Edward Kuczaj. 'It Just Happened': Looking at Crime Events, Marian Liebmann. 9. Art Therapy with Homeless People, Claire Swainson.

**Introducing Network Analysis
in Social Work**
Philip Seed
1989 ISBN 1 85302 024 9
This textbook is designed for social workers
and others in social work practice as a guide
to the application of a systematic method for
understanding and using social networks.

Social Work and Health Care
Edited by Rex Taylor and Jill Ford
1989 ISBN 1 85302 016 8
The book reviews the problems and opportunities for joint work in the interface between social work and health care.

**Social Work Management
and Practice: Systems Principles**
Sue Ross and Andy Bilson
1989 ISBN 1 85302 022 2
The authors look at the whole basis of social
work intervention and address the question of
how change can usefully be brought about
with individual clients and within agencies,
suggesting key principles for effective social
work within a systems framework.

Why Day Care?
Edited by Gordon Horobin
1987 ISBN 1 85302 000 1

**Living with Mental Handicap:
Transitions in the Lives of People
with Mental Handicap**
Edited by Gordon Horobin and David May
1988 ISBN 1 85302 004 4

**Developing Services for the Elderly
2nd edition**
Edited by Joyce Lishman and
Gordon Horobin
1985 ISBN 1 85091 003 0

Responding to Mental Illness
Edited by Gordon Horobin
1985 ISBN 1 85091 005 7

Evaluation 2nd edition
Edited by Joyce Lishman
1988 ISBN 1 85302 006 0

Approaches to Addiction
Edited by Joyce Lishman
and Gordon Horobin
1985 ISBN 1 85091 001 4

**Community Care: Strategy
for Improvement**
The Private Care Sector Alternative
1988 ISBN 1 85302 X

**New Information Technology
in Management and Practice**
Edited by Gordon Horobin
and Stuart Montgomery
1986 ISBN 1 85091 022 7

**Health Services Privatization
in Industrial Societies**
Edited by Joseph L Scarpaci
1990 ISBN 1 85302 064 8
This book is the first to look at the theory and
practice of privatization of health services in-
ternationally. The contributors provide original case studies of privatization in Great
Britain, West Germany, Sweden, France,
New Zealand, the United States, Canada, and
Chile. Among the sectors of health care they
examine are public and private hospitals, environmental health programmes to prevent
cancer, mental health care, prepaid health
plans, and the multinational pharmaceutical
industry. Writing from the vantage point of
medical geography, they demonstrate how
the restructuring of health care systems affects local communities in markedly uneven
ways.
Ultimately, Scarpaci and the contributors
conclude, conflicts arising from economic
and geographic inequities implicit in privatization will limit the degree to which any government can dismantle its health care
services.